THE VEGETARIAN DIET FOR BEGINNERS

Cookbook

100+ Super Easy Recipes to Start a **Healthier** Lifestyle! The **Best Recipes** You Need to Jump into the **Tastiest Plant-Based** World!

By

Jocelyn Grant

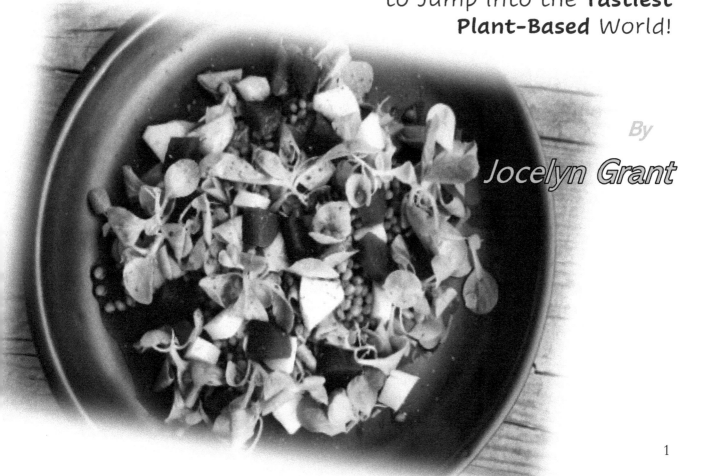

Table of Contents

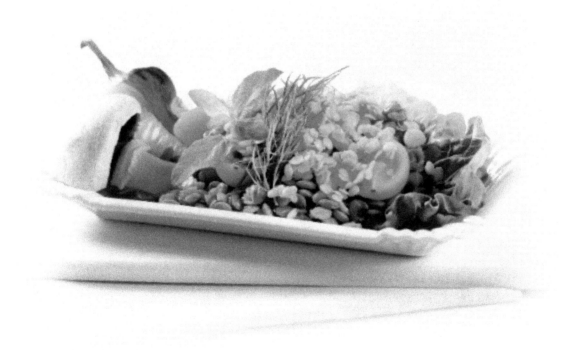

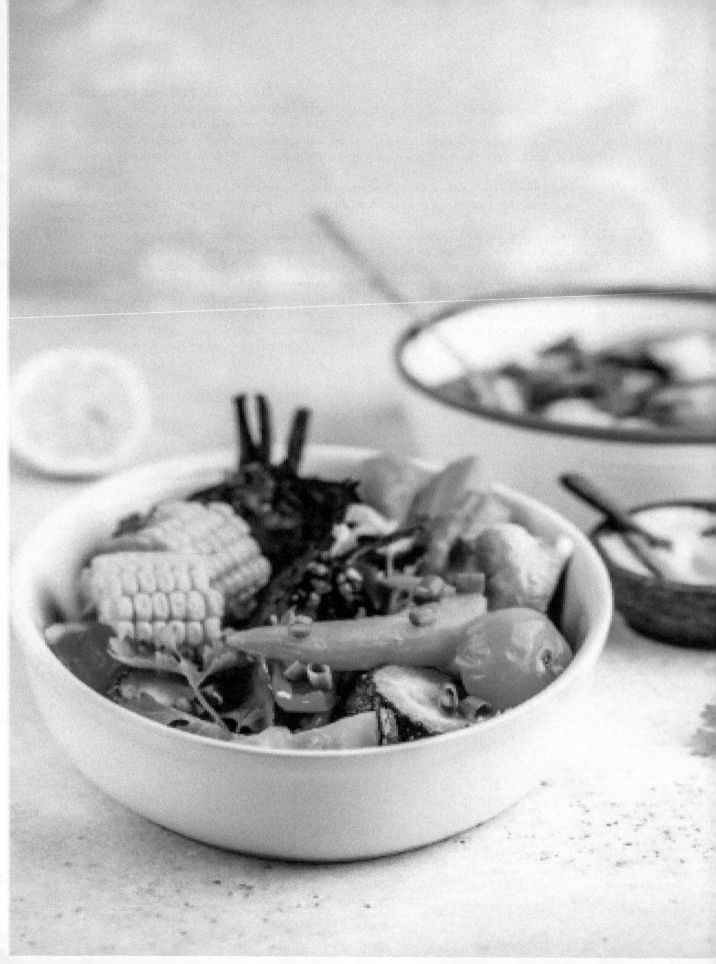

Introduction

The **Vegetarian** diet allows you to get the right amount of nutrients and follow a meal plan that makes you light and fit!

In the latest years, people have been thinking more and more about what they eat: they are concerned about eating healthy foods to provide the right nutrients to the body, but they are also interested in eating meals that are no full of preservatives or additives. People are increasingly concerned with eating less processed and more sustainable foods and this trend has turned many people into vegetarians or even vegans.
And the plant-based diet is really the best solution!

The vegetarian diet is suitable for everyone: **children**, **people over 50**, **athletes**, **women**, **men** and it is easy to learn even for **beginners**!

Especially a beginner could learn the basics of Vegetarian Diet having the right information! And… what is no better than a simple-to-follow cookbook with the simplest **100** Vegetarian recipes?

In "Vegetarian Diet for Beginners *Cookbook*", you will find only simple and quick recipes to have healthy meals!

Ready to discover the best 100 Vegetarian Recipes? LET'S GO!

Chapter 1.
BREAKFAST AND SNACKS

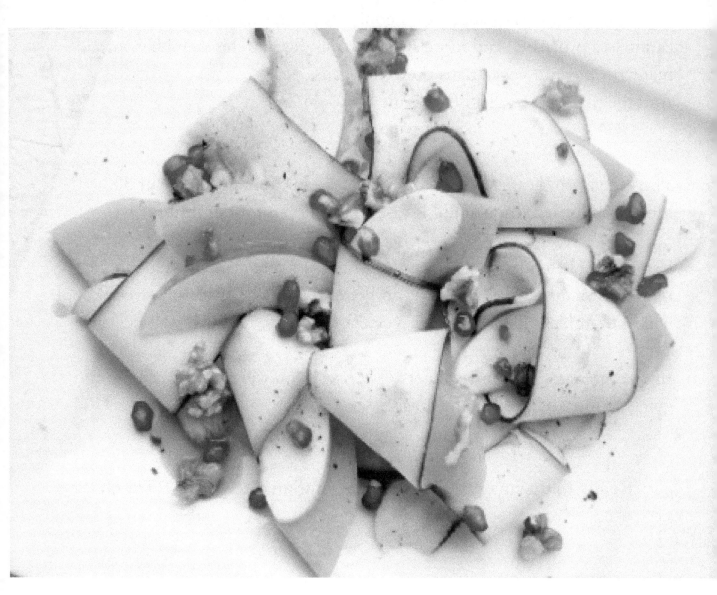

1) ITALIAN MUSHROOM AND SPINACH CHICKPEA OMELETTE

Preparation Time: 25 minutes | | **Servings: 4**

Ingredients:

- ✓ 1 cup chickpea flour
- ✓ ½ tsp onion powder
- ✓ ½ tsp garlic powder
- ✓ ¼ tsp white pepper
- ✓ 1/3 cup nutritional yeast
- ✓ ½ tsp baking soda
- ✓ 1 green bell pepper, chopped

- ✓ 3 scallions, chopped
- ✓ 1 cup sautéed button mushrooms
- ✓ ½ cup chopped fresh spinach
- ✓ 1 cup halved cherry tomatoes
- ✓ 1 tbsp fresh parsley leaves

Directions:

❖ In a medium bowl, mix the chickpea flour, onion powder, garlic powder, white pepper, nutritional yeast, and baking soda until well combined. Heat a medium skillet over medium heat and add a quarter of the batter. Swirl the pan to spread the batter across the pan. Scatter a quarter each of the bell pepper, scallions, mushrooms, and spinach on top and cook until the bottom part of the omelet sets, 1-2 minutes.

❖ Carefully flip the omelet and cook the other side until set and golden brown. Transfer the omelet to a plate and make the remaining omelets. Serve the omelet with the tomatoes and garnish with the parsley leaves

2) EXOTIC COCONUT-RASPBERRY PANCAKES

Preparation Time: 25 minutes | | **Servings: 4**

Ingredients:

- ✓ 2 tbsp flax seed powder
- ✓ ½ cup coconut milk
- ✓ ¼ cup fresh raspberries, mashed
- ✓ ½ cup oat flour
- ✓ 1 tsp baking soda
- ✓ A pinch salt
- ✓ 1 tbsp coconut sugar

- ✓ 2 tbsp pure date syrup
- ✓ ½ tsp cinnamon powder
- ✓ 2 tbsp unsweetened coconut flakes
- ✓ 2 tsp plant butter
- ✓ Fresh raspberries for garnishing

Directions:

❖ In a medium bowl, mix the flax seed powder with the 6 tbsp water and thicken for 5 minutes. Mix in coconut milk and raspberries. Add the oat flour, baking soda, salt, coconut sugar, date syrup, and cinnamon powder. Fold in the coconut flakes until well combined.

❖ Working in batches, melt a quarter of the butter in a non-stick skillet and add ¼ cup of the batter. Cook until set beneath and golden brown, 2 minutes. Flip the pancake and cook on the other side until set and golden brown, 2 minutes. Transfer to a plate and make the remaining pancakes using the rest of the ingredients in the same proportions. Garnish the pancakes with some raspberries and serve warm

3) ENGLISH BLUEBERRY-CHIA PUDDING

Preparation Time: 5 minutes + chilling time | | **Servings: 2**

Ingredients:

- ✓ ¾ cup coconut milk
- ✓ ½ tsp vanilla extract
- ✓ ½ cup blueberries

- ✓ 2 tbsp chia seeds
- ✓ Chopped walnuts to garnish

Directions:

❖ In a blender, pour the coconut milk, vanilla extract, and half of the blueberries. Process the ingredients at high speed until the blueberries have incorporated into the liquid.

❖ Open the blender and mix in the chia seeds. Share the mixture into two breakfast jars, cover, and refrigerate for 4 hours to allow the mixture to gel. Garnish the pudding with the remaining blueberries and walnuts. Serve immediately

9

4) EASY POTATO AND CAULIFLOWER BROWNS

Preparation Time: 35 minutes		Servings: 4

Ingredients:

- ✓ 3 tbsp flax seed powder
- ✓ 2 large potatoes, shredded
- ✓ 1 big head cauliflower, riced
- ✓ ½ white onion, grated
- ✓ Salt and black pepper to taste
- ✓ 4 tbsp plant butter

Directions:

❖ In a medium bowl, mix the flaxseed powder and 9 tbsp water. Allow thickening for 5 minutes for the vegan "flax egg." Add the potatoes, cauliflower, onion, salt, and black pepper to the vegan "flax egg" and mix until well combined. Allow sitting for 5 minutes to thicken.

❖ Working in batches, melt 1 tbsp of plant butter in a non-stick skillet and add 4 scoops of the hashbrown mixture to the skillet. Make sure to have 1 to 2-inch intervals between each scoop.

❖ Use the spoon to flatten the batter and cook until compacted and golden brown on the bottom part, 2 minutes. Flip the hashbrowns and cook further for 2 minutes or until the vegetable cook and is golden brown. Transfer to a paper-towel-lined plate to drain grease. Make the remaining hashbrowns using the remaining ingredients. Serve warm

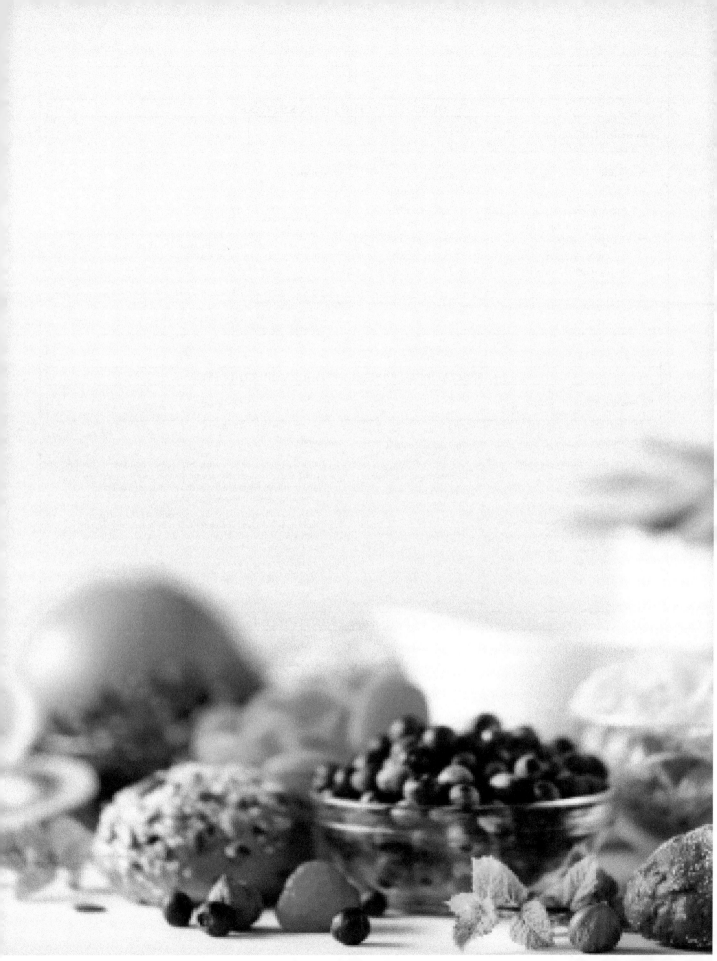

5) QUICK PISTACHIOS-PUMPKIN CAKE

Preparation Time: 70 minutes		Servings: 4

Ingredients:

- ✓ 2 tbsp flaxseed powder
- ✓ 3 tbsp vegetable oil
- ✓ ¾ cup canned pumpkin puree
- ✓ ½ cup pure corn syrup
- ✓ 3 tbsp pure date sugar
- ✓ 1 ½ cups whole-wheat flour
- ✓ ½ tsp cinnamon powder
- ✓ ½ tsp baking powder
- ✓ ¼ tsp cloves powder
- ✓ ½ tsp allspice powder
- ✓ ½ tsp nutmeg powder
- ✓ 2 tbsp chopped pistachios

Directions:

- ❖ Preheat the oven to 350 F and lightly coat an 8 x 4-inch loaf pan with cooking spray. In a bowl, mix the flax seed powder with 6 tbsp water and allow thickening for 5 minutes to make the vegan "flax egg."
- ❖ In a bowl, whisk the vegetable oil, pumpkin puree, corn syrup, date sugar, and vegan "flax egg." In another bowl, mix the flour, cinnamon powder, baking powder, cloves powder, allspice powder, and nutmeg powder. Add this mixture to the wet batter and mix until well combined. Pour the batter into the loaf pan, sprinkle the pistachios on top, and gently press the nuts onto the batter to stick.
- ❖ Bake in the oven for 50-55 minutes or until a toothpick inserted into the cake comes out clean. Remove the cake onto a wire rack, allow cooling, slice, and serve

6) SPECIAL BELL PEPPER WITH SCRAMBLED TOFU

Preparation Time: 20 minutes		Servings: 4

Ingredients:

- ✓ 2 tbsp plant butter, for frying
- ✓ 1 (14 oz) pack firm tofu, crumbled
- ✓ 1 red bell pepper, chopped
- ✓ 1 green bell pepper, chopped
- ✓ 1 tomato, finely chopped
- ✓ 2 tbsp chopped fresh green onions
- ✓ Salt and black pepper to taste
- ✓ 1 tsp turmeric powder
- ✓ 1 tsp Creole seasoning
- ✓ ½ cup chopped baby kale
- ✓ ¼ cup grated plant-based Parmesan

Directions:

- ❖ Melt the plant butter in a skillet over medium heat and add the tofu. Cook with occasional stirring until the tofu is light golden brown while, making sure not to break the tofu into tiny bits but to have scrambled egg resemblance, 5 minutes.
- ❖ Stir in the bell peppers, tomato, green onions, salt, black pepper, turmeric powder, and Creole seasoning. Sauté until the vegetables soften, 5 minutes. Mix in the kale to wilt, 3 minutes and then half of the plant-based Parmesan cheese.
- ❖ Allow melting for 1 to 2 minutes and then turn the heat off. Top with the remaining cheese and serve warm

7) TRADITIONAL FRENCH TOAST

Preparation Time: 20 minutes		Servings: 2

Ingredients:

- ✓ 1 tbsp ground flax seeds
- ✓ 1 cup coconut milk
- ✓ 1/2 tsp vanilla paste
- ✓ A pinch of sea salt
- ✓ A pinch of grated nutmeg
- ✓ 1/2 tsp ground cinnamon
- ✓ 1/4 tsp ground cloves
- ✓ 1 tbsp agave syrup
- ✓ 4 slices bread

Directions:

- ❖ In a mixing bowl, thoroughly combine the flax seeds, coconut milk, vanilla, salt, nutmeg, cinnamon, cloves and agave syrup.
- ❖ Dredge each slice of bread into the milk mixture until well coated on all sides.
- ❖ Preheat an electric griddle to medium heat and lightly oil it with a nonstick cooking spray.
- ❖ Cook each slice of bread on the preheated griddle for about 3 minutes per side until golden brown.
- ❖ Enjoy

8) CRISPY FRYBREAD WITH PEANUT BUTTER AND JAM

Preparation Time: 20 minutes | | **Servings: 3**

Ingredients:

- ✓ 1 cup all-purpose flour
- ✓ 1/2 tsp baking powder
- ✓ 1/2 tsp sea salt
- ✓ 1 tsp coconut sugar
- ✓ 1/2 cup warm water
- ✓ 3 tsp olive oil
- ✓ 3 tbsp peanut butter
- ✓ 3 tbsp raspberry jam

Directions:

- ❖ Thoroughly combine the flour, baking powder, salt and sugar. Gradually add in the water until the dough comes together.
- ❖ Divide the dough into three balls; flatten each ball to create circles.
- ❖ Heat 1 tsp of the olive oil in a frying pan over a moderate flame. Fry the first bread for about 9 minutes or until golden brown. Repeat with the remaining oil and dough.
- ❖ Serve the frybread with the peanut butter and raspberry jam. Enjoy

9) EASY PUDDING WITH SULTANAS ON CIABATTA BREAD

Preparation Time: 2 hours 10 minutes | | **Servings: 4**

Ingredients:

- ✓ 2 cups coconut milk, unsweetened
- ✓ 1/2 cup agave syrup
- ✓ 1 tbsp coconut oil
- ✓ 1/2 tsp vanilla essence
- ✓ 1/2 tsp ground cardamom
- ✓ 1/4 tsp ground cloves
- ✓ 1/2 tsp ground cinnamon
- ✓ 1/4 tsp Himalayan salt
- ✓ 3/4 pound stale ciabatta bread, cubed
- ✓ 1/2 cup sultana raisins

Directions:

- ❖ In a mixing bowl, combine the coconut milk, agave syrup, coconut oil, vanilla, cardamom, ground cloves, cinnamon and Himalayan salt.
- ❖ Add the bread cubes to the custard mixture and stir to combine well. Fold in the sultana raisins and allow it to rest for about 1 hour on a counter.
- ❖ Then, spoon the mixture into a lightly oiled casserole dish.
- ❖ Bake in the preheated oven at 350 degrees F for about 1 hour or until the top is golden brown.
- ❖ Place the bread pudding on a wire rack for 10 minutes before slicing and serving

10) VEGAN FRIENDLY BANH MI

Preparation Time: 35 minutes | | **Servings: 4**

Ingredients:
- ✓ 1/2 cup rice vinegar
- ✓ 1/4 cup water
- ✓ 1/4 cup white sugar
- ✓ 2 carrots, cut into 1/16-inch-thick matchsticks
- ✓ 1/2 cup white (daikon) radish, cut into 1/16-inch-thick matchsticks
- ✓ 1 white onion, thinly sliced
- ✓ 2 tbsp olive oil
- ✓ 12 ounces firm tofu, cut into sticks
- ✓ 1/4 cup vegan mayonnaise
- ✓ 1 ½ tbsp soy sauce
- ✓ 2 cloves garlic, minced
- ✓ 1/4 cup fresh parsley, chopped
- ✓ Kosher salt and ground black pepper, to taste
- ✓ 2 standard French baguettes, cut into four pieces
- ✓ 4 tbsp fresh cilantro, chopped
- ✓ 4 lime wedges

Directions:
- ❖ Bring the rice vinegar, water and sugar to a boil and stir until the sugar has dissolved, about 1 minute. Allow it to cool.
- ❖ Pour the cooled vinegar mixture over the carrot, daikon radish and onion; allow the vegetables to marinate for at least 30 minutes.
- ❖ While the vegetables are marinating, heat the olive oil in a frying pan over medium-high heat. Once hot, add the tofu and sauté for 8 minutes, stirring occasionally to promote even cooking.
- ❖ Then, mix the mayo, soy sauce, garlic, parsley, salt and ground black pepper in a small bowl.
- ❖ Slice each piece of the baguette in half the long way Then, toast the baguette halves under the preheated broiler for about 3 minutes.
- ❖ To assemble the banh mi sandwiches, spread each half of the toasted baguette with the mayonnaise mixture; fill the cavity of the bottom half of the bread with the fried tofu sticks, marinated vegetables and cilantro leaves.
- ❖ Lastly, squeeze the lime wedges over the filling and top with the other half of the baguette. Enjoy

11) EASY BREAKFAST NUTTY OATMEAL MUFFINS

Preparation Time: 30 minutes | | **Servings:** 9

Ingredients:

- ✓ 1 ½ cups rolled oats
- ✓ 1/2 cup shredded coconut, unsweetened
- ✓ 3/4 tsp baking powder
- ✓ 1/4 tsp salt
- ✓ 1/4 tsp vanilla extract
- ✓ 1/4 tsp coconut extract
- ✓ 1/4 tsp grated nutmeg
- ✓ 1/2 tsp cardamom
- ✓ 3/4 cup coconut milk
- ✓ 1/3 cup canned pumpkin
- ✓ 1/4 cup agave syrup
- ✓ 1/4 cup golden raisins
- ✓ 1/4 cup pecans, chopped

Directions:

- ❖ Begin by preheating your oven to 360 degrees F. Spritz a muffin tin with a nonstick cooking oil.
- ❖ In a mixing bowl, thoroughly combine all the ingredients, except for the raisins and pecans.
- ❖ Fold in the raisins and pecans and scrape the batter into the prepared muffin tin.
- ❖ Bake your muffins for about 25 minutes or until the top is set. Enjoy

12) SPECIAL SMOOTHIE BOWL OF RASPBERRY AND CHIA

Preparation Time: 10 minutes | | **Servings:** 2

Ingredients:

- ✓ 1 cup coconut milk
- ✓ 2 small-sized bananas, peeled
- ✓ 1 ½ cups raspberries, fresh or frozen
- ✓ 2 dates, pitted
- ✓ 1 tbsp coconut flakes
- ✓ 1 tbsp pepitas
- ✓ 2 tbsp chia seeds

Directions:

- ❖ In your blender or food processor, mix the coconut milk with the bananas, raspberries and dates.
- ❖ Process until creamy and smooth. Divide the smoothie between two bowls.
- ❖ Top each smoothie bowl with the coconut flakes, pepitas and chia seeds. Enjoy

13) ORIGINAL BREAKFAST OATS WITH WALNUTS AND CURRANTS

Preparation Time: 10 minutes | | **Servings:** 2

Ingredients:

- ✓ 1 cup water
- ✓ 1 ½ cups oat milk
- ✓ 1 ½ cups rolled oats
- ✓ A pinch of salt
- ✓ A pinch of grated nutmeg
- ✓ 1/4 tsp cardamom
- ✓ 1 handful walnuts, roughly chopped
- ✓ 4 tbsp dried currants

Directions:

- ❖ In a deep saucepan, bring the water and milk to a rolling boil. Add in the oats, cover the saucepan and turn the heat to medium.
- ❖ Add in the salt, nutmeg and cardamom. Continue to cook for about 12 to 13 minutes more, stirring occasionally.
- ❖ Spoon the mixture into serving bowls; top with walnuts and currants. Enjoy

14) SWEET APPLESAUCE PANCAKES WITH COCONUT

Preparation Time: 50 minutes		**Servings: 8**

Ingredients:

- ✓ 1 ¼ cups whole-wheat flour
- ✓ 1 tsp baking powder
- ✓ 1/4 tsp sea salt
- ✓ 1/2 tsp coconut sugar
- ✓ 1/4 tsp ground cloves
- ✓ 1/4 tsp ground cardamom
- ✓ 1/2 tsp ground cinnamon
- ✓ 3/4 cup oat milk
- ✓ 1/2 cup applesauce, unsweetened
- ✓ 2 tbsp coconut oil
- ✓ 8 tbsp coconut, shredded
- ✓ 8 tbsp pure maple syrup

Directions:

- ❖ In a mixing bowl, thoroughly combine the flour, baking powder, salt, sugar and spices. Gradually add in the milk and applesauce.
- ❖ Heat a frying pan over a moderately high flame and add a small amount of the coconut oil.
- ❖ Once hot, pour the batter into the frying pan. Cook for approximately 3 minutes until the bubbles form; flip it and cook on the other side for 3 minutes longer until browned on the underside. Repeat with the remaining oil and batter.
- ❖ Serve with shredded coconut and maple syrup. Enjoy

15) LOVELY VEGGIE PANINI

Preparation Time: 30 minutes		**Servings: 4**

Ingredients:

- ✓ 1 tbsp olive oil
- ✓ 1 cup sliced button mushrooms
- ✓ Salt and black pepper to taste
- ✓ 1 ripe avocado, sliced
- ✓ 2 tbsp freshly squeezed lemon juice
- ✓ 1 tbsp chopped parsley
- ✓ ½ tsp pure maple syrup
- ✓ 8 slices whole-wheat ciabatta
- ✓ 4 oz sliced plant-based Parmesan

Directions:

- ❖ Heat the olive oil in a medium skillet over medium heat and sauté the mushrooms until softened, 5 minutes. Season with salt and black pepper. Turn the heat off.
- ❖ Preheat a panini press to medium heat, 3 to 5 minutes. Mash the avocado in a medium bowl and mix in the lemon juice, parsley, and maple syrup. Spread the mixture on 4 bread slices, divide the mushrooms and plant-based Parmesan cheese on top.
- ❖ Cover with the other bread slices and brush the top with olive oil. Grill the sandwiches one after another in the heated press until golden brown, and the cheese is melted.
- ❖ Serve

16) SIMPLE ORANGE CREPES

Preparation Time: 30 minutes		Servings: 4

Ingredients:

- ✓ 2 tbsp flax seed powder
- ✓ 1 tsp vanilla extract
- ✓ 1 tsp pure date sugar
- ✓ ¼ tsp salt

- ✓ 2 cups almond flour
- ✓ 1 ½ cups oat milk
- ✓ ½ cup melted plant butter
- ✓ 3 tbsp fresh orange juice
- ✓ 3 tbsp plant butter for frying

Directions:

- ❖ In a medium bowl, mix the flax seed powder with 6 tbsp water and allow thickening for 5 minutes to make the vegan "flax egg." Whisk in the vanilla, date sugar, and salt.
- ❖ Pour in a quarter cup of almond flour and whisk, then a quarter cup of oat milk, and mix until no lumps remain. Repeat the mixing process with the remaining almond flour and almond milk in the same quantities until exhausted.
- ❖ Mix in the plant butter, orange juice, and half of the water until the mixture is runny like pancakes. Add the remaining water until the mixture is lighter. Brush a non-stick skillet with some butter and place over medium heat to melt.
- ❖ Pour 1 tbsp of the batter into the pan and swirl the skillet quickly and all around to coat the pan with the batter. Cook until the batter is dry and golden brown beneath, about 30 seconds.
- ❖ Use a spatula to flip the crepe and cook the other side until golden brown too. Fold the crepe onto a plate and set aside. Repeat making more crepes with the remaining batter until exhausted. Drizzle some maple syrup on the crepes and serve

17) ENGLISH OAT BREAD WITH COCONUT

Preparation Time: 50 minutes		Servings: 4

Ingredients:

- ✓ 4 cups whole-wheat flour
- ✓ ¼ tsp salt
- ✓ ½ cup rolled oats

- ✓ 1 tsp baking soda
- ✓ 1 ¾ cups coconut milk, thick
- ✓ 2 tbsp pure maple syrup

Directions:

- ❖ Preheat the oven to 400 F.
- ❖ In a bowl, mix flour, salt, oats, and baking soda. Add in coconut milk and maple syrup and whisk until dough forms. Dust your hands with some flour and knead the dough into a ball. Shape the dough into a circle and place on a baking sheet.
- ❖ Cut a deep cross on the dough and bake in the oven for 15 minutes at 450 F. Reduce the temperature to 400 F and bake further for 20 to 25 minutes or until a hollow sound is made when the bottom of the bread is tapped. Slice and serve

18) MEXICAN BOWL WITH BLACK BEANS AND SPICY QUINOA

Preparation Time: 25 minutes		Servings: 4

Ingredients:

- ✓ 1 cup brown quinoa, rinsed
- ✓ 3 tbsp plant-based yogurt
- ✓ ½ lime, juiced
- ✓ 2 tbsp chopped fresh cilantro
- ✓ 1 (5 oz) can black beans, drained
- ✓ 3 tbsp tomato salsa
- ✓ ¼ avocado, sliced
- ✓ 2 radishes, shredded
- ✓ 1 tbsp pepitas (pumpkin seeds)

Directions:

- ❖ Cook the quinoa with 2 cups of slightly salted water in a medium pot over medium heat or until the liquid absorbs, 15 minutes. Spoon the quinoa into serving bowls and fluff with a fork.
- ❖ In a small bowl, mix the yogurt, lime juice, cilantro, and salt. Divide this mixture on the quinoa and top with the beans, salsa, avocado, radishes, and pepitas. Serve immediately

19) ITALIAN ALMOND AND RAISIN GRANOLA

Preparation Time: 20 minutes		Servings: 8

Ingredients:

- ✓ 5 ½ cups old-fashioned oats
- ✓ 1 ½ cups chopped walnuts
- ✓ ½ cup shelled sunflower seeds
- ✓ 1 cup golden raisins
- ✓ 1 cup shaved almonds
- ✓ 1 cup pure maple syrup
- ✓ ½ tsp ground cinnamon
- ✓ ¼ tsp ground allspice
- ✓ A pinch of salt

Directions:

- ❖ Preheat oven to 325 F. In a baking dish, place the oats, walnuts, and sunflower seeds. Bake for 10 minutes.
- ❖ Lower the heat from the oven to 300 F. Stir in the raisins, almonds, maple syrup, cinnamon, allspice, and salt. Bake for an additional 15 minutes. Allow cooling before serving

Chapter 2. LUNCH

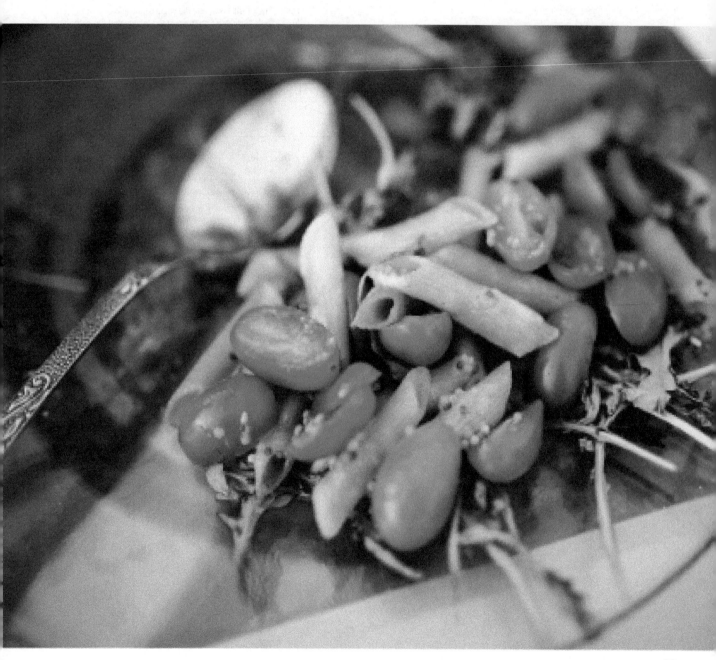

20) SPECIAL BEAN AND PECAN SANDWICHES

Preparation Time: 20 minutes		Servings: 4

Ingredients:

- ✓ 1 onion, chopped
- ✓ 1 garlic clove, crushed
- ✓ ¾ cup pecans, chopped
- ✓ ¾ cup canned black beans
- ✓ ¾ cup almond flour
- ✓ 2 tbsp minced fresh parsley
- ✓ 1 tbsp soy sauce
- ✓ 1 tsp Dijon mustard + to serve
- ✓ Salt and black pepper to taste
- ✓ ½ tsp ground sage
- ✓ ½ tsp sweet paprika
- ✓ 2 tbsp olive oil
- ✓ Bread slices
- ✓ Lettuce leaves and sliced tomatoes

Directions:

❖ Put the onion, garlic, and pecans in a blender and pulse until roughly ground. Add in the beans and pulse until everything is well combined. Transfer to a large mixing bowl and stir in the flour, parsley, soy sauce, mustard, salt, sage, paprika, and pepper. Mold patties out of the mixture.

❖ Heat the oil in a skillet over medium heat. Brown the patties for 10 minutes on both sides. To assemble, lay patties on the bread slices and top with mustard, lettuce, and tomato slices

21) SIMPLE HOMEMADE KITCHARI

Preparation Time: 40 minutes		Servings: 5

Ingredients:

- ✓ 4 cups chopped cauliflower and broccoli florets
- ✓ ½ cup split peas
- ✓ ½ cup brown rice
- ✓ 1 red onion, chopped
- ✓ 1 (14.5-oz) can diced tomatoes
- ✓ 3 garlic cloves, minced
- ✓ 1 jalapeño pepper, seeded
- ✓ ½ tsp ground ginger
- ✓ 1 tsp ground turmeric
- ✓ 1 tsp olive oil
- ✓ 1 tsp fennel seeds
- ✓ Juice of 1 large lemon
- ✓ Salt and black pepper to taste

Directions:

❖ In a food processor, place the onion, tomatoes with juices, garlic, jalapeño pepper, ginger, turmeric, and 2 tbsp of water. Pulse until ingredients are evenly mixed.

❖ Heat the oil in a pot over medium heat. Cook the cumin and fennel seeds for 2-3 minutes, stirring often. Pour in the puréed mixture, split peas, rice, and 3 cups of water. Bring to a boil, then lower the heat and simmer for 10 minutes. Stir in cauliflower, broccoli, and cook for another 10 minutes. Mix in lemon juice and adjust seasoning

22) PICCANTE GREEN RICE

Preparation Time: 35 minutes		Servings: 4

Ingredients:

- ✓ 1 roasted bell pepper, chopped
- ✓ 3 small hot green chilies, chopped
- ✓ 2 ½ cups vegetable broth
- ✓ ½ cup chopped fresh parsley
- ✓ 1 onion, chopped
- ✓ 2 garlic cloves, chopped
- ✓ Salt and black pepper to taste
- ✓ ½ tsp dried oregano
- ✓ 3 tbsp canola oil
- ✓ 1 cup long-grain brown rice
- ✓ 1 ½ cups cooked black beans
- ✓ 2 tbsp minced fresh cilantro

Directions:

❖ In a food processor, place bell pepper, chilies, 1 cup of broth, parsley, onion, garlic, pepper, oregano, salt, and pepper and blend until smooth. Heat oil in a skillet over medium heat. Add in rice and veggie mixture. Cook for 5 minutes, stirring often. Add in the remaining broth and bring to a boil, lower the heat, and simmer for 15 minutes. Mix in beans and cook for another 5 minutes. Serve with cilantro

23) SPECIAL ASIAN QUINOA SAUTÉ

Preparation Time: 30 minutes		Servings: 4

Ingredients:

- ✓ 1 cup quinoa
- ✓ Salt to taste
- ✓ 1 head cauliflower, break into florets
- ✓ 2 tsp untoasted sesame oil
- ✓ 1 cup snow peas, cut in half
- ✓ 1 cup frozen peas
- ✓ 2 cups chopped Swiss chard
- ✓ 2 scallions, chopped
- ✓ 2 tbsp water
- ✓ 1 tsp toasted sesame oil
- ✓ 1 tbsp soy sauce
- ✓ 2 tbsp sesame seeds

Directions:

- ❖ Place quinoa with 2 cups of water and salt in a bowl. Bring to a boil, lower the heat and simmer for 15 minutes. Do not stir.
- ❖ Heat the oil in a skillet over medium heat and sauté the cauliflower for 4-5 minutes. Add in snow peas and stir well. Stir in Swiss chard, scallions, and 2 tbsp of water; cook until wilted, about 5 minutes. Season with salt.
- ❖ Drizzle with sesame oil and soy sauce and cook for 1 minute. Divide the quinoa in bowls and top with the cauliflower mixture. Garnish with sesame seeds and soy sauce to serve

24) ITALIAN FARRO AND BLACK BEAN LOAF

Preparation Time: 50 minutes		Servings: 6

Ingredients:

- ✓ 3 tbsp olive oil
- ✓ 1 onion, minced
- ✓ 1 cup faro
- ✓ 2 (15.5-oz) cans black beans, mashed
- ✓ ½ cup quick-cooking oats
- ✓ 1/3 cup whole-wheat flour
- ✓ 2 tbsp nutritional yeast
- ✓ 1 ½ tsp dried thyme
- ✓ ½ tsp dried oregano

Directions:

- ❖ Heat the oil in a pot over medium heat. Place in onion and sauté for 3 minutes. Add in faro, 2 cups of water, salt, and pepper. Bring to a boil, lower the heat and simmer for 20 minutes. Remove to a bowl.
- ❖ Preheat oven to 350 F.
- ❖ Add the mashed beans, oats, flour, yeast, thyme, and oregano to the faro bowl. Toss to combine. Taste and adjust the seasoning. Shape the mixture into a greased loaf. Bake for 20 minutes. Let cool for a few minutes. Slice and serve

25) SPECIAL CUBAN-STYLE MILLET

Preparation Time: 40 minutes		Servings: 4

Ingredients:

- ✓ 2 tbsp olive oil
- ✓ 1 onion, chopped
- ✓ 2 zucchinis, chopped
- ✓ 2 garlic cloves, minced
- ✓ 1 tsp dried thyme
- ✓ ½ tsp ground cumin
- ✓ 1 (15.5-oz) can black-eyed peas
- ✓ 1 cup millet
- ✓ 2 tbsp chopped fresh cilantro

Directions:

- ❖ Heat the oil in a pot over medium heat. Place in onion and sauté for 3 minutes until translucent. Add in zucchinis, garlic, thyme, and cumin and cook for 10 minutes. Put in peas, millet, and 2 ½ cups of hot water. Bring to a boil, then lower the heat and simmer for 20 minutes. Fluff the millet using a fork. Serve garnished with cilantro

26) CLASSIC CILANTRO PILAF

Preparation Time: 30 minutes		Servings: 6

Ingredients:

- ✓ 3 tbsp olive oil
- ✓ 1 onion, minced
- ✓ 1 carrot, chopped
- ✓ 2 garlic cloves, minced
- ✓ 1 cup wild rice
- ✓ 1 ½ tsp ground fennel seeds
- ✓ ½ tsp ground cumin
- ✓ Salt and black pepper to taste
- ✓ 3 tbsp minced fresh cilantro

Directions:

❖ Heat the oil in a pot over medium heat. Place in onion, carrot, and garlic and sauté for 5 minutes. Stir in rice, fennel seeds, cumin, and 2 cups water. Bring to a boil, then lower the heat and simmer for 20 minutes. Remove to a bowl and fluff using a fork. Serve topped with cilantro and black pepper

27) TYPICAL ORIENTAL BULGUR ANDWHITE BEANS

Preparation Time: 55 minutes		Servings: 4

Ingredients:

- ✓ 2 tbsp olive oil
- ✓ 3 green onions, chopped
- ✓ 1 cup bulgur
- ✓ 1 cups water
- ✓ 1 tbsp soy sauce
- ✓ Salt to taste
- ✓ 1 ½ cups cooked white beans
- ✓ 1 tbsp nutritional yeast
- ✓ 1 tbsp dried parsley

Directions:

❖ Heat the oil in a pot over medium heat. Place in green onions and sauté for 3 minutes. Stir in bulgur, water, soy sauce, and salt. Bring to a boil, then lower the heat and simmer for 20-22 minutes. Mix in beans and yeast. Cook for 5 minutes. Serve topped with parsley

28) RED LENTILS WITH MUSHROOMS

Preparation Time: 25 minutes		Servings: 4

Ingredients:

- ✓ 2 tsp olive oil
- ✓ 2 cloves garlic, minced
- ✓ 2 tsp grated fresh ginger
- ✓ ½ tsp ground cumin
- ✓ ½ tsp fennel seeds
- ✓ 1 cup mushrooms, chopped
- ✓ 1 large tomato, chopped
- ✓ 1 cup dried red lentils
- ✓ 2 tbsp lemon juice

Directions:

❖ Heat the oil in a pot over medium heat. Place in the garlic and ginger and cook for 3 minutes. Stir in cumin, fennel, mushrooms, tomato, lentils, and 2 ¼ cups of water. Bring to a boil, then lower the heat and simmer for 15 minutes. Mix in lemon juice and serve

29) SPECIAL COLORFUL RISOTTO WITH VEGETABLES

Preparation Time: 35 minutes		Servings: 5

Ingredients:

- ✓ 2 tbsp sesame oil
- ✓ 1 onion, chopped
- ✓ 2 bell peppers, chopped
- ✓ 1 parsnip, trimmed and chopped
- ✓ 1 carrot, trimmed and chopped
- ✓ 1 cup broccoli florets
- ✓ 2 garlic cloves, finely chopped
- ✓ 1/2 tsp ground cumin
- ✓ 2 cups brown rice
- ✓ Sea salt and black pepper, to taste
- ✓ 1/2 tsp ground turmeric
- ✓ 2 tbsp fresh cilantro, finely chopped

Directions:

❖ Heat the sesame oil in a saucepan over medium-high heat.
❖ Once hot, cook the onion, peppers, parsnip, carrot and broccoli for about 3 minutes until aromatic.
❖ Add in the garlic and ground cumin; continue to cook for 30 seconds more until aromatic.
❖ Place the brown rice in a saucepan and cover with cold water by 2 inches. Bring to a boil. Turn the heat to a simmer and continue to cook for about 30 minutes or until tender.
❖ Stir the rice into the vegetable mixture; season with salt, black pepper and ground turmeric; garnish with fresh cilantro and serve immediately. Enjoy

30) EASY AMARANT GRITS WITH WALNUTS

Preparation Time: 35 minutes		Servings: 4

Ingredients:

- ✓ 2 cups water
- ✓ 2 cups coconut milk
- ✓ 1 cup amaranth
- ✓ 1 cinnamon stick
- ✓ 1 vanilla bean
- ✓ 4 tbsp maple syrup
- ✓ 4 tbsp walnuts, chopped

Directions:

- ❖ Bring the water and coconut milk to a boil over medium-high heat; add in the amaranth, cinnamon and vanilla and turn the heat to a simmer.
- ❖ Let it cook for about 30 minutes, stirring periodically to prevent the amaranth from sticking to the bottom of the pan.
- ❖ Top with maple syrup and walnuts. Enjoy

31) DELICIOUS BARLEY PILAF WITH WILD MUSHROOMS

Preparation Time: 45 minutes		Servings: 4

Ingredients:

- ✓ 2 tbsp vegan butter
- ✓ 1 small onion, chopped
- ✓ 1 tsp garlic, minced
- ✓ 1 jalapeno pepper, seeded and minced
- ✓ 1 pound wild mushrooms, sliced
- ✓ 1 cup medium pearl barley, rinsed
- ✓ 2 ¾ cups vegetable broth

Directions:

- ❖ Melt the vegan butter in a saucepan over medium-high heat.
- ❖ Once hot, cook the onion for about 3 minutes until just tender.
- ❖ Add in the garlic, jalapeno pepper, mushrooms; continue to sauté for 2 minutes or until aromatic.
- ❖ Add in the barley and broth, cover and continue to simmer for about 30 minutes. Once all the liquid has absorbed, allow the barley to rest for about 10 minutes fluff with a fork.
- ❖ Taste and adjust the seasonings. Enjoy

32) ITALIAN POLENTA WITH MUSHROOMS AND CHICKPEAS

Preparation Time: 25 minutes		Servings: 4

Ingredients:

- ✓ 3 cups vegetable broth
- ✓ 1 cup yellow cornmeal
- ✓ 2 tbsp olive oil
- ✓ 1 onion, chopped
- ✓ 1 bell pepper, seeded and sliced
- ✓ 1 pound Cremini mushrooms, sliced
- ✓ 2 garlic cloves, minced
- ✓ 1/2 cup dry white wine
- ✓ 1/2 cup vegetable broth
- ✓ Kosher salt and freshly ground black pepper, to taste
- ✓ 1 tsp paprika
- ✓ 1 cup canned chickpeas, drained

Directions:

- ❖ In a medium saucepan, bring the vegetable broth to a boil over medium-high heat. Now, add in the cornmeal, whisking continuously to prevent lumps.
- ❖ Reduce the heat to a simmer. Continue to simmer, whisking periodically, for about 18 minutes, until the mixture has thickened.
- ❖ Meanwhile, heat the olive oil in a saucepan over a moderately high heat. Cook the onion and pepper for about 3 minutes or until just tender and fragrant.
- ❖ Add in the mushrooms and garlic; continue to sauté, gradually adding the wine and broth, for 4 more minutes or until cooked through. Season with salt, black pepper and paprika. Stir in the chickpeas.
- ❖ Spoon the mushroom mixture over your polenta and serve warm. Enjoy

33) HEALTHY TEFF SALAD WITH AVOCADO AND BEANS

Preparation Time: 20 minutes + chilling time		Servings: 2

Ingredients:

- ✓ 2 cups water
- ✓ 1/2 cup teff grain
- ✓ 1 tsp fresh lemon juice
- ✓ 3 tbsp vegan mayonnaise
- ✓ 1 tsp deli mustard
- ✓ 1 small avocado, pitted, peeled and sliced
- ✓ 1 small red onion, thinly sliced
- ✓ 1 small Persian cucumber, sliced
- ✓ 1/2 cup canned kidney beans, drained
- ✓ 2 cups baby spinach

Directions:

- ❖ In a deep saucepan, bring the water to a boil over high heat. Add in the teff grain and turn the heat to a simmer.
- ❖ Continue to cook, covered, for about 20 minutes or until tender. Let it cool completely.
- ❖ Add in the remaining ingredients and toss to combine. Serve at room temperature. Enjoy

34) ENGLISH OVERNIGHT OATMEAL WITH WALNUTS

Preparation Time: 5 minutes + chilling time		Servings: 3

Ingredients:

- ✓ 1 cup old-fashioned oats
- ✓ 3 tbsp chia seeds
- ✓ 1 ½ cups coconut milk
- ✓ 3 tsp agave syrup
- ✓ 1 tsp vanilla extract
- ✓ 1/2 tsp ground cinnamon
- ✓ 3 tbsp walnuts, chopped
- ✓ A pinch of salt
- ✓ A pinch of grated nutmeg

Directions:

- ❖ Divide the ingredients between three mason jars.
- ❖ Cover and shake to combine well. Let them sit overnight in your refrigerator.
- ❖ You can add some extra milk before serving. Enjoy

35) HEALTHY AND COLORFUL SPELT SALAD

Preparation Time: 50 minutes + chilling time		Servings: 4

Ingredients:

- ✓ 3 ½ cups water
- ✓ 1 cup dry spelt
- ✓ 1 cup canned kidney beans, drained
- ✓ 1 bell pepper, seeded and diced
- ✓ 2 medium tomatoes, diced
- ✓ 2 tbsp basil, chopped
- ✓ 2 tbsp parsley, chopped
- ✓ 2 tbsp mint, chopped
- ✓ 1/4 cup extra-virgin olive oil
- ✓ 1 tsp deli mustard
- ✓ 1 tbsp fresh lime juice
- ✓ 1 tbsp white vinegar
- ✓ Sea salt and cayenne pepper, to taste

Directions:

- ❖ Bring the water to a boil over medium-high heat. Now, add in the spelt, turn the heat to a simmer and continue to cook for approximately 50 minutes, until the spelt is tender. Drain and allow it to cool completely.
- ❖ Toss the spelt with the remaining ingredients; toss to combine well and place the salad in your refrigerator until ready to serve.
- ❖ Enjoy

36) EASY POWERFUL TEFF BOWL WITH TAHINI SAUCE

Preparation Time: 20 minutes + chilling time		Servings: 4

Ingredients:

- ✓ 3 cups water
- ✓ 1 cup teff
- ✓ 2 garlic cloves, pressed
- ✓ 4 tbsp tahini
- ✓ 2 tbsp tamari sauce
- ✓ 2 tbsp white vinegar
- ✓ 1 tsp agave nectar
- ✓ 1 tsp deli mustard
- ✓ 1 tsp Italian herb mix
- ✓ 1 cup canned chickpeas, drained
- ✓ 2 cups mixed greens
- ✓ 1 cup grape tomatoes, halved
- ✓ 1 Italian peppers, seeded and diced

Directions:

- ❖ In a deep saucepan, bring the water to a boil over high heat. Add in the teff grain and turn the heat to a simmer.
- ❖ Continue to cook, covered, for about 20 minutes or until tender. Let it cool completely and transfer to a salad bowl.
- ❖ In the meantime, mix the garlic, tahini, tamari sauce, vinegar, agave nectar, mustard and Italian herb mix; whisk until everything is well incorporated.
- ❖ Add the canned chickpeas, mixed greens, tomatoes and peppers to the salad bowl; toss to combine. Dress the salad and toss again. Serve at room temperature. Enjoy

37) ITALIAN POLENTA TOASTS WITH BALSAMIC ONIONS

Preparation Time: 25 minutes + chilling time		Servings: 5

Ingredients:
- ✓ 3 cups vegetable broth
- ✓ 1 cup yellow cornmeal
- ✓ 4 tbsp vegan butter, divided
- ✓ 2 tbsp olive oil
- ✓ 2 large onions, sliced
- ✓ Sea salt and ground black pepper, to taste
- ✓ 1 thyme sprig, chopped
- ✓ 1 tbsp balsamic vinegar

Directions:
- ❖ In a medium saucepan, bring the vegetable broth to a boil over medium-high heat. Now, add in the cornmeal, whisking continuously to prevent lumps.
- ❖ Reduce the heat to a simmer. Continue to simmer, whisking periodically, for about 18 minutes, until the mixture has thickened. Stir the vegan butter into the cooked polenta.
- ❖ Spoon the cooked polenta into a lightly greased square baking dish. Cover with the plastic wrap and chill for about 2 hours or until firm.
- ❖ Meanwhile, heat the olive oil in a nonstick skillet over a moderately high heat. Cook the onions for about 3 minutes or until just tender and fragrant.
- ❖ Stir in the salt, black pepper, thyme and balsamic vinegar and continue to sauté for 1 minute or so; remove from the heat.
- ❖ Cut your polenta into squares. Spritz a nonstick skillet with a cooking spray. Fry the polenta squares for about 5 minutes per side or until golden brown.
- ❖ Top each polenta toast with the balsamic onion and serve. Enjoy

38) SPECIAL FREEKEH PILAF WITH CHICKPEAS

Preparation Time: 40 minutes		Servings: 4

Ingredients:

- ✓ 4 tbsp olive oil
- ✓ 1 cup shallots, chopped
- ✓ 1 celery stalks, chopped
- ✓ 1 carrot, chopped
- ✓ 1 tsp garlic, minced
- ✓ Sea salt and ground black pepper, to taste
- ✓ 1 tsp cayenne pepper
- ✓ 1 tsp dried basil
- ✓ 1 tsp dried oregano
- ✓ 1 cup freekeh
- ✓ 2 ½ cups water
- ✓ 1 cup boiled chickpeas, drained
- ✓ 2 tbsp roasted peanuts, roughly chopped
- ✓ 2 tbsp fresh mint, roughly chopped

Directions:

- ❖ Heat the olive oil in a heavy-bottomed pot over medium-high heat. Once hot, sauté the shallot, celery and carrot for about 3 minutes until just tender.
- ❖ Then, add in the garlic and continue to sauté for 30 seconds more or until aromatic. Add in the spices, freekeh and water.
- ❖ Turn the heat to a simmer for 30 to 35 minutes, stirring occasionally to promote even cooking. Fold in the boiled chickpeas.
- ❖ To serve, spoon into individual bowls and garnish with roasted peanuts and fresh mint. Enjoy

39) BEST ITALIAN RICE WITH BROCCOLI

Preparation Time: 30 minutes		Servings: 4

Ingredients:

- ✓ 2 tbsp olive oil
- ✓ 1 shallot, chopped
- ✓ 1 tsp ginger, minced
- ✓ 1 tsp garlic, minced
- ✓ 1/2 pound broccoli florets
- ✓ 1 cup Arborio rice
- ✓ 4 cups roasted vegetable broth

Directions:

- ❖ In a medium-sized pot, heat the olive oil over a moderately high flame. Add in the shallot and cook for about 3 minutes or until tender and translucent.
- ❖ Then, add in the ginger and garlic and continue to cook for 30 seconds more. Add in the broccoli and rice and continue to cook for 4 minutes more.
- ❖ Pour the vegetable broth into the saucepan and bring to a boil; immediately turn the heat to a gentle simmer.
- ❖ Cook for about 20 minutes or until all the liquid has absorbed. Taste and adjust the seasonings. Enjoy

40) ENGLISH OVERNIGHT OATMEAL WITH PRUNES

Preparation Time: 5 minutes + chilling time		Servings: 2

Ingredients:

- ✓ 1 cup hemp milk
- ✓ 1 tbsp flax seed, ground
- ✓ 2/3 cup rolled oats
- ✓ 2 ounces prunes, sliced
- ✓ 2 tbsp agave syrup
- ✓ A pinch of salt
- ✓ 1/2 tsp ground cinnamon

Directions:

- ❖ Divide the ingredients, except for the prunes, between two mason jars.
- ❖ Cover and shake to combine well. Let them sit overnight in your refrigerator.
- ❖ Garnish with sliced prunes just before serving. Enjoy

41) SWEET MINI CORNBREAD PUDDINGS

Preparation Time: 30 minutes		Servings: 8

Ingredients:

- ✓ 1 cup all-purpose flour
- ✓ 1 cup yellow cornmeal
- ✓ 1 tsp baking powder
- ✓ 1 tsp baking soda
- ✓ 1 tsp sea salt
- ✓ 2 tbsp brown sugar
- ✓ 1/2 tsp ground allspice
- ✓ 1 cup soy yogurt
- ✓ 1/4 cup vegan butter, melted
- ✓ 1 tsp apple cider vinegar
- ✓ 1 red bell pepper, seeded and chopped
- ✓ 1 green bell pepper, seeded and chopped
- ✓ 1 cup marinated mushrooms, chopped
- ✓ 2 small pickled cucumbers, chopped
- ✓ 1 tbsp fresh basil, chopped
- ✓ 1 tbsp fresh cilantro, chopped
- ✓ 1 tbsp fresh chives, chopped

Directions:

- ❖ Start by preheating your oven to 420 degrees F. Now, spritz a muffin tin with a non-stick cooking spray.
- ❖ In a mixing bowl, thoroughly combine the flour, cornmeal, baking soda, baking powder, salt, sugar and ground allspice.
- ❖ Gradually add in the yogurt, vegan butter and apple cider vinegar, whisking constantly to avoid lumps. Fold in the vegetables and herbs.
- ❖ Scrape the batter into the prepared muffin tin. Bake your muffins for about 25 minutes or until a toothpick inserted in the middle comes out dry and clean.
- ❖ Transfer them to a wire rack to rest for 5 minutes before unmolding and serving. Enjoy

42) LOVELY SHERRY SHALLOT BEANS

Preparation Time: 25 minutes		**Servings: 4**

Ingredients:

- ✓ 2 tsp olive oil
- ✓ 4 shallots, chopped
- ✓ 1 tsp ground cumin
- ✓ 1 (14.5-oz) cans black beans
- ✓ 1 cup vegetable broth
- ✓ 2 tbsp sherry vinegar

Directions:

- ❖ Heat the oil in a pot over medium heat. Place in shallots and cumin and cook for 3 minutes until soft. Stir in beans and broth. Bring to a boil, then lower the heat and simmer for 10 minutes. Add in sherry vinegar, increase the heat and cook for an additional 3 minutes. Serve warm

43) SIMPLE QUINOA AND CHICKPEA POT

Preparation Time: 15 minutes		**Servings: 2**

Ingredients:

- ✓ 2 tsp olive oil
- ✓ 1 cup cooked quinoa
- ✓ 1 (15-oz) can chickpeas
- ✓ 1 bunch arugula chopped
- ✓ 1 tbsp soy
- ✓ Sea salt and black pepper to taste

Directions:

- ❖ Heat the oil in a skillet over medium heat. Stir in quinoa, chickpeas, and arugula and cook for 3-5 minutes until the arugula wilts. Pour in soy sauce, salt, and pepper. Toss to coat. Serve immediately

44) EVERYDAY BUCKWHEAT PILAF WITH PINE NUTS

Preparation Time: 25 minutes		**Servings: 4**

Ingredients:

- ✓ 1 cup buckwheat groats
- ✓ 2 cups vegetable stock
- ✓ ¼ cup pine nuts
- ✓ 2 tbsp olive oil
- ✓ ½ onion, chopped
- ✓ ⅓ cup chopped fresh parsley

Directions:

- ❖ Put the groats and vegetable stock in a pot. Bring to a boil, then lower the heat and simmer for 15 minutes. Heat a skillet over medium heat. Place in the pine nuts and toast for 2-3 minutes, shaking often. Heat the oil in the same skillet and sauté the onion for 3 minutes until translucent.
- ❖ Once the groats are ready, fluff them using a fork. Mix in pine nuts, onion, and parsley. Sprinkle with salt and pepper. Serve

45)

45) ITALIAN HOLIDAY STUFFING

Preparation Time: 25 minutes		**Servings: 4**

Ingredients:

- ✓ ¼ cup plant butter
- ✓ 1 onion, chopped
- ✓ 2 celery stalks, sliced
- ✓ 1 cup button mushrooms, sliced
- ✓ 3 garlic cloves, minced
- ✓ ½ cup vegetable broth
- ✓ ½ cup raisins
- ✓ ½ cup chopped walnuts
- ✓ 2 cups cooked quinoa
- ✓ 1 tsp Italian seasoning
- ✓ Sea salt to taste
- ✓ Chopped fresh parsley

Directions:

- ❖ In a skillet over medium heat, melt the butter. Sauté the onion, garlic, celery, and mushrooms for 5 minutes until tender, stirring occasionally. Pour in broth, raisins, and walnuts. Bring to a boil, then lower the heat and simmer for 5 minutes. Stir in quinoa, Italian seasoning, and salt. Cook for another 4 minutes. Serve garnished with parsley

46) SPECIAL PRESSURE COOKER GREEN LENTILS

Preparation Time: 30 minutes		Servings: 6

Ingredients:

- ✓ 3 tbsp coconut oil
- ✓ 2 tbsp curry powder
- ✓ 1 tsp ground ginger
- ✓ 1 onion, chopped
- ✓ 2 garlic cloves, sliced
- ✓ 1 cup dried green lentils
- ✓ 3 cups water
- ✓ Salt and black pepper to taste

Directions:

- ❖ Set your IP to Sauté. Add in coconut oil, curry powder, ginger, onion, and garlic. Cook for 3 minutes. Stir in green lentils. Pour in water. Lock the lid and set the time to 10 minutes on High. Once ready, perform a natural pressure release for 10 minutes. Unlock the lid and season with salt and pepper. Serve

47) SUPER CHERRY AND PISTACHIO BULGUR

Preparation Time: 45 minutes		Servings: 4

Ingredients:

- ✓ 1 tbsp plant butter
- ✓ 1 white onion, chopped
- ✓ 1 carrot, chopped
- ✓ 1 celery stalk, chopped
- ✓ 1 cup chopped mushrooms
- ✓ 1 ½ cups bulgur
- ✓ 4 cups vegetable broth
- ✓ 1 cup chopped dried cherries, soaked
- ✓ ½ cup chopped pistachios

Directions:

- ❖ Preheat oven to 375 F.
- ❖ Melt butter in a skillet over medium heat. Sauté the onion, carrot, and celery for 5 minutes until tender. Add in mushrooms and cook for 3 more minutes. Pour in bulgur and broth. Transfer to a casserole and bake covered for 30 minutes. Once ready, uncover and stir in cherries. Top with pistachios to serve

48) EVERYDAY MUSHROOM FRIED RICE

Preparation Time: 25 minutes		Servings: 6

Ingredients:

- ✓ 2 tbsp sesame oil
- ✓ 1 onion, chopped
- ✓ 1 carrot, chopped
- ✓ 1 cup okra, chopped
- ✓ 1 cup sliced shiitake mushrooms
- ✓ 2 garlic cloves, minced
- ✓ ¼ cup soy sauce
- ✓ 1 cups cooked brown rice
- ✓ 2 green onions, chopped

Directions:

- ❖ Heat the oil in a skillet over medium heat. Place in onion and carrot and cook for 3 minutes. Add in okra and mushrooms, cook for 5-7 minutes. Stir in garlic and cook for 30 seconds. Put in soy sauce and rice. Cook until hot. Add in green onions and stir. Serve warm

49) BEST BEAN AND BROWN RICE WITH ARTICHOKES

Preparation Time: 35 minutes		Servings: 4

Ingredients:

- ✓ 2 tbsp olive oil
- ✓ 3 garlic cloves, minced
- ✓ 1 cup artichokes hearts, chopped
- ✓ 1 tsp dried basil
- ✓ 1 ½ cups cooked navy beans
- ✓ 1 ½ cups long-grain brown rice
- ✓ 3 cups vegetable broth
- ✓ Salt and black pepper to taste
- ✓ 2 ripe grape tomatoes, quartered
- ✓ 2 tbsp minced fresh parsley

Directions:

- ❖ Heat the oil in a pot over medium heat. Sauté the garlic for 1 minute. Stir in artichokes, basil, navy beans, rice, and broth. Sprinkle with salt and pepper. Lower the heat and simmer for 20-25 minutes. Remove to a bowl and mix in tomatoes and parsley. Using a fork, fluff the rice and serve right away

50) SPECIAL PRESSURE COOKER CELERY AND SPINACH CHICKPEAS

Preparation Time: 50 minutes		Servings: 5

Ingredients:

- ✓ 1 cup chickpeas, soaked overnight
- ✓ 1 onion, chopped
- ✓ 2 garlic cloves, minced
- ✓ 1 celery stalk, chopped
- ✓ 2 tbsp olive oil
- ✓ 3 tsp ground cinnamon
- ✓ ½ tsp ground nutmeg
- ✓ 1 tbsp coconut oil
- ✓ 1 cup spinach, chopped

Directions:

- ❖ Place chickpeas in your IP with the onion, garlic, celery, olive oil, 2 cups water, cinnamon, and nutmeg.
- ❖ Lock the lid in place; set the time to 30 minutes on High. Once ready, perform a natural pressure release for 10 minutes. Unlock the lid and drain the excess water. Put back the chickpeas and stir in coconut oil and spinach. Set the pot to Sauté and cook for another 5 minutes

51) VEGGIE SPANISH PAELLA WITH LENTILS

Preparation Time: 50 minutes		Servings: 4

Ingredients:

- ✓ 2 tbsp olive oil
- ✓ 1 onion, chopped
- ✓ 1 green bell pepper, chopped
- ✓ 2 garlic cloves, minced
- ✓ 1 (14.5-oz) can diced tomatoes
- ✓ 1 tbsp capers
- ✓ ¼ tsp crushed red pepper
- ✓ 1 ½ cups long-grain brown rice
- ✓ 3 cups vegetable broth
- ✓ 1 ½ cups cooked lentils, drained
- ✓ ¼ cup sliced pitted black olives
- ✓ 2 tbsp minced fresh parsley

Directions:

- ❖ Heat oil in a pot over medium heat and sauté onion, bell pepper, and garlic for 5 minutes. Stir in tomatoes, capers, red pepper, and salt. Cook for 5 minutes. Pour in the rice and broth. Bring to a boil, then lower the heat. Simmer for 20 minutes. Turn the heat off and mix in lentils. Serve garnished with olives and parsley

Chapter 3. DINNER

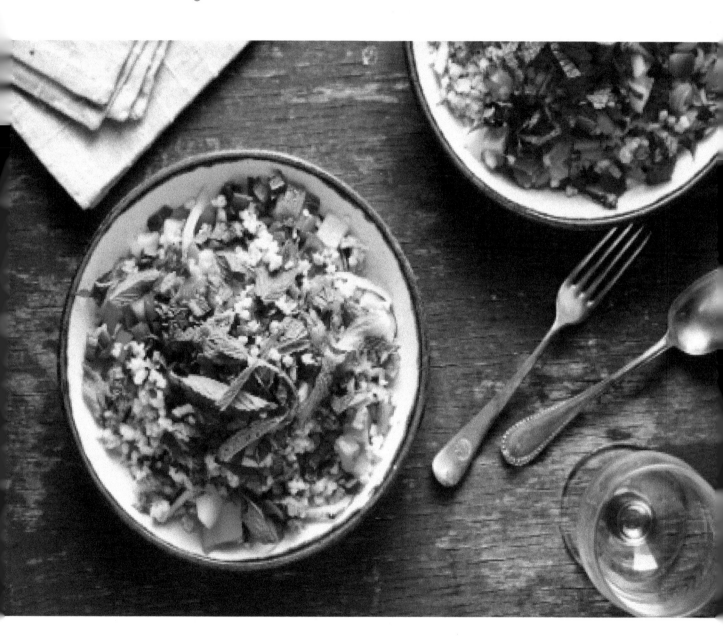

52) DELICIOUS SWEET AND SPICY BRUSSEL SPROUT STIR-FRY

Preparation Time: 15 minutes

Servings: 4

Ingredients:

- ✓ 4 oz plant butter + more to taste
- ✓ 4 shallots, chopped
- ✓ 1 tbsp apple cider vinegar
- ✓ Salt and black pepper to taste
- ✓ 1 lb Brussels sprouts
- ✓ Hot chili sauce

Directions:

- ❖ Put the plant butter in a saucepan and melt over medium heat. Pour in the shallots and sauté for 2 minutes, to caramelize and slightly soften. Add the apple cider vinegar, salt, and black pepper. Stir and reduce the heat to cook the shallots further with continuous stirring, about 5 minutes. Transfer to a plate after.
- ❖ Trim the Brussel sprouts and cut in halves. Leave the small ones as wholes. Pour the Brussel sprouts into the saucepan and stir-fry with more plant butter until softened but al dente. Season with salt and black pepper, stir in the onions and hot chili sauce, and heat for a few seconds. Serve immediately

53) MEXICAN BLACK BEAN BURGERS WITH BBQ SAUCE

Preparation Time: 20 minutes

Servings: 4

Ingredients:

- ✓ 3 (15 oz) cans black beans, drained
- ✓ 2 tbsp whole-wheat flour
- ✓ 2 tbsp quick-cooking oats
- ✓ ¼ cup chopped fresh basil
- ✓ 2 tbsp pure barbecue sauce
- ✓ 1 garlic clove, minced
- ✓ Salt and black pepper to taste
- ✓ 4 whole-grain hamburger buns, split
- ✓ For topping:
- ✓ Red onion slices
- ✓ Tomato slices
- ✓ Fresh basil leaves
- ✓ Additional barbecue sauce

Directions:

- ❖ In a medium bowl, mash the black beans and mix in the flour, oats, basil, barbecue sauce, garlic salt, and black pepper until well combined. Mold 4 patties out of the mixture and set aside.
- ❖ Heat a grill pan to medium heat and lightly grease with cooking spray. Cook the bean patties on both sides until light brown and cooked through, 10 minutes. Place the patties between the burger buns and top with the onions, tomatoes, basil, and some barbecue sauce. Serve warm

54) LOVELY CREAMY BRUSSELS SPROUTS BAKE

Preparation Time: 26 minutes

Servings: 4

Ingredients:

- ✓ 3 tbsp plant butter
- ✓ 1 cup tempeh, cut into 1-inch cubes
- ✓ 1 ½ lb halved Brussels sprouts
- ✓ 5 garlic cloves, minced
- ✓ 1 ¼ cups coconut cream
- ✓ 10 oz grated plant-based mozzarella
- ✓ ¼ cup grated plant-based Parmesan
- ✓ Salt and black pepper to taste

Directions:

- ❖ Preheat oven to 400 F.
- ❖ Melt the plant butter in a large skillet over medium heat and fry the tempeh cubes until browned on both sides, about 6 minutes. Remove onto a plate and set aside. Pour the Brussels sprouts and garlic into the skillet and sauté until fragrant.
- ❖ Mix in coconut cream and simmer for 4 minutes. Add tempeh cubes and combine well. Pour the sauté into a baking dish, sprinkle with plant-based mozzarella cheese, and plant-based Parmesan cheese. Bake for 10 minutes or until golden brown on top. Serve with tomato salad

55) GENOVESE BASIL PESTO SEITAN PANINI

Preparation Time: 15 minutes+ cooling time | | **Servings: 4**

Ingredients:

- ✓ For the seitan:
- ✓ 2/3 cup basil pesto
- ✓ ½ lemon, juiced
- ✓ 1 garlic clove, minced
- ✓ 1/8 tsp salt
- ✓ 1 cup chopped seitan

- ✓ For the panini:
- ✓ 3 tbsp basil pesto
- ✓ 8 thick slices whole-wheat ciabatta
- ✓ Olive oil for brushing
- ✓ 8 slices plant-based mozzarella
- ✓ 1 yellow bell pepper, chopped
- ✓ ¼ cup grated plant Parmesan cheese

Directions:

- ❖ In a medium bowl, mix the pesto, lemon juice, garlic, and salt. Add the seitan and coat well with the marinade. Cover with plastic wrap and marinate in the refrigerator for 30 minutes.
- ❖ Preheat a large skillet over medium heat and remove the seitan from the fridge. Cook the seitan in the skillet until brown and cooked through, 2-3 minutes. Turn the heat off.
- ❖ Preheat a panini press to medium heat. In a small bowl, mix the pesto in the inner parts of two slices of bread. On the outer parts, apply some olive oil and place a slice with (the olive oil side down) in the press. Lay 2 slices of plant-based mozzarella cheese on the bread, spoon some seitan on top. Sprinkle with some bell pepper and some plant-based Parmesan cheese. Cover with another bread slice.
- ❖ Close the press and grill the bread for 1 to 2 minutes. Flip the bread, and grill further for 1 minute or until the cheese melts and golden brown on both sides. Serve warm

56) ENGLISH SWEET OATMEAL "GRITS"

Preparation Time: 20 minutes | | **Servings: 4**

Ingredients:

- ✓ 1 ½ cups steel-cut oats, soaked overnight
- ✓ 1 cup almond milk
- ✓ 2 cups water
- ✓ A pinch of grated nutmeg

- ✓ A pinch of ground cloves
- ✓ A pinch of sea salt
- ✓ 4 tbsp almonds, slivered
- ✓ 6 dates, pitted and chopped
- ✓ 6 prunes, chopped

Directions:

- ❖ In a deep saucepan, bring the steel cut oats, almond milk and water to a boil.
- ❖ Add in the nutmeg, cloves and salt. Immediately turn the heat to a simmer, cover and continue to cook for about 15 minutes or until they've softened.
- ❖ Then, spoon the grits into four serving bowls; top them with the almonds, dates and prunes.
- ❖ Enjoy!

57) SPECIAL FREEKEH BOWL WITH DRIED FIGS

Preparation Time: 35 minutes | | **Servings: 2**

Ingredients:

- ✓ 1/2 cup freekeh, soaked for 30 minutes, drained
- ✓ 1 1/3 cups almond milk
- ✓ 1/4 tsp sea salt

- ✓ 1/4 tsp ground cloves
- ✓ 1/4 tsp ground cinnamon
- ✓ 4 tbsp agave syrup
- ✓ 2 ounces dried figs, chopped

Directions:

- ❖ Place the freekeh, milk, sea salt, ground cloves and cinnamon in a saucepan. Bring to a boil over medium-high heat.
- ❖ Immediately turn the heat to a simmer for 30 to 35 minutes, stirring occasionally to promote even cooking.
- ❖ Stir in the agave syrup and figs. Ladle the porridge into individual bowls and serve. Enjoy

58) EASY CORNMEAL PORRIDGE WITH MAPLE SYRUP

Preparation Time: 20 minutes		Servings: 4

Ingredients:

- ✓ 2 cups water
- ✓ 2 cups almond milk
- ✓ 1 cinnamon stick
- ✓ 1 vanilla bean
- ✓ 1 cup yellow cornmeal
- ✓ 1/2 cup maple syrup

Directions:

- ❖ In a saucepan, bring the water and almond milk to a boil. Add in the cinnamon stick and vanilla bean.
- ❖ Gradually add in the cornmeal, stirring continuously; turn the heat to a simmer. Let it simmer for about 15 minutes.
- ❖ Drizzle the maple syrup over the porridge and serve warm. Enjoy

59) ITALIAN AROMATIC MILLET BOWL

Preparation Time: 20 minutes		Servings: 3

Ingredients:

- ✓ 1 cup water
- ✓ 1 ½ cups coconut milk
- ✓ 1 cup millet, rinsed and drained
- ✓ 1/4 tsp crystallized ginger
- ✓ 1/4 tsp ground cinnamon
- ✓ A pinch of grated nutmeg
- ✓ A pinch of Himalayan salt
- ✓ 2 tbsp maple syrup

Directions:

- ❖ Place the water, milk, millet, crystallized ginger cinnamon, nutmeg and salt in a saucepan; bring to a boil.
- ❖ Turn the heat to a simmer and let it cook for about 20 minutes; fluff the millet with a fork and spoon into individual bowls.
- ❖ Serve with maple syrup. Enjoy

60) SPICY HARISSA BULGUR BOWL

Preparation Time: 25 minutes		Servings: 4

Ingredients:

- ✓ 1 cup bulgur wheat
- ✓ 1 ½ cups vegetable broth
- ✓ 2 cups sweet corn kernels, thawed
- ✓ 1 cup canned kidney beans, drained
- ✓ 1 red onion, thinly sliced
- ✓ 1 garlic clove, minced
- ✓ Sea salt and ground black pepper, to taste
- ✓ 1/4 cup harissa paste
- ✓ 1 tbsp lemon juice
- ✓ 1 tbsp white vinegar
- ✓ 1/4 cup extra-virgin olive oil
- ✓ 1/4 cup fresh parsley leaves, roughly chopped

Directions:

- ❖ In a deep saucepan, bring the bulgur wheat and vegetable broth to a simmer; let it cook, covered, for 12 to 13 minutes.
- ❖ Let it stand for 5 to 10 minutes and fluff your bulgur with a fork.
- ❖ Add the remaining ingredients to the cooked bulgur wheat; serve warm or at room temperature. Enjoy

61) EXOTIC COCONUT QUINOA PUDDING

Preparation Time: 20 minutes		Servings: 3

Ingredients:

- ✓ 1 cup water
- ✓ 1 cup coconut milk
- ✓ 1 cup quinoa
- ✓ A pinch of kosher salt
- ✓ A pinch of ground allspice
- ✓ 1/2 tsp cinnamon
- ✓ 1/2 tsp vanilla extract
- ✓ 4 tbsp agave syrup
- ✓ 1/2 cup coconut flakes

Directions:

- ❖ Place the water, coconut milk, quinoa, salt, ground allspice, cinnamon and vanilla extract in a saucepan.
- ❖ Bring it to a boil over medium-high heat. Turn the heat to a simmer and let it cook for about 20 minutes; fluff with a fork and add in the agave syrup.
- ❖ Divide between three serving bowls and garnish with coconut flakes. Enjoy

62) ITALIAN CREMINI MUSHROOM RISOTTO

Preparation Time: 20 minutes		**Servings: 3**

Ingredients:

- ✓ 3 tbsp vegan butter
- ✓ 1 tsp garlic, minced
- ✓ 1 tsp thyme
- ✓ 1 pound Cremini mushrooms, sliced
- ✓ 1 ½ cups white rice
- ✓ 2 ½ cups vegetable broth
- ✓ 1/4 cup dry sherry wine
- ✓ Kosher salt and ground black pepper, to taste
- ✓ 3 tbsp fresh scallions, thinly sliced

Directions:

- ❖ In a saucepan, melt the vegan butter over a moderately high flame. Cook the garlic and thyme for about 1 minute or until aromatic.
- ❖ Add in the mushrooms and continue to sauté until they release the liquid or about 3 minutes.
- ❖ Add in the rice, vegetable broth and sherry wine. Bring to a boil; immediately turn the heat to a gentle simmer.
- ❖ Cook for about 15 minutes or until all the liquid has absorbed. Fluff the rice with a fork, season with salt and pepper and garnish with fresh scallions. Enjoy

63) MEXICAN-STYLE JALAPEÑO QUINOA BOWL WITH LIMA BEANS

Preparation Time: 30 minutes		**Servings: 4**

Ingredients:

- ✓ 1 tbsp olive oil
- ✓ 1 lb extra firm tofu, cubed
- ✓ Salt and black pepper to taste
- ✓ 1 medium yellow onion, finely diced
- ✓ ½ cup cauliflower florets
- ✓ 1 jalapeño pepper, minced
- ✓ 2 garlic cloves, minced
- ✓ 1 tbsp red chili powder
- ✓ 1 tsp cumin powder
- ✓ 1 (8 oz) can sweet corn kernels
- ✓ 1 (8 oz) can lima beans, rinsed
- ✓ 1 cup quick-cooking quinoa
- ✓ 1 (14 oz) can diced tomatoes
- ✓ 2 ½ cups vegetable broth
- ✓ 1 cup grated plant-based cheddar
- ✓ 2 tbsp chopped fresh cilantro
- ✓ 2 limes, cut into wedges
- ✓ 1 avocado, pitted, sliced, and peeled

Directions:

- ❖ Heat olive oil in a pot and cook the tofu until golden brown, 5 minutes. Season with salt, pepper, and mix in onion, cauliflower, and jalapeño pepper. Cook until the vegetables soften, 3 minutes.
- ❖ Stir in garlic, chili powder, and cumin powder; cook for 1 minute. Mix in sweet corn kernels, lima beans, quinoa, tomatoes, and vegetable broth. Simmer until the quinoa absorbs all the liquid, 10 minutes. Fluff quinoa. Top with the plant-based cheddar cheese, cilantro, lime wedges, and avocado. Serve

64) SIMPLE PAN-FRIED ASPARAGUS

Preparation Time: 10 minutes		**Servings: 4**

Ingredients:

- ✓ 4 tbsp vegan butter
- ✓ 1 ½ pounds asparagus spears, trimmed
- ✓ 1/2 tsp cumin seeds, ground
- ✓ 1/4 tsp bay leaf, ground
- ✓ Sea salt and ground black pepper, to taste
- ✓ 1 tsp fresh lime juice

Directions:

- ❖ Melt the vegan butter in a saucepan over medium-high heat.
- ❖ Sauté the asparagus for about 3 to 4 minutes, stirring periodically to promote even cooking.
- ❖ Add in the cumin seeds, bay leaf, salt and black pepper and continue to cook the asparagus for 2 minutes more until crisp-tender.
- ❖ Drizzle lime juice over the asparagus and serve warm. Enjoy

65) EASY GINGERY CARROT MASH

Preparation Time: 25 minutes | | **Servings: 4**

Ingredients:

- ✓ 2 pounds carrots, cut into rounds
- ✓ 2 tbsp olive oil
- ✓ 1 tsp ground cumin
- ✓ Salt ground black pepper, to taste
- ✓ 1/2 tsp cayenne pepper
- ✓ 1/2 tsp ginger, peeled and minced
- ✓ 1/2 cup whole milk

Directions:

- ❖ Begin by preheating your oven to 400 degrees F.
- ❖ Toss the carrots with the olive oil, cumin, salt, black pepper and cayenne pepper. Arrange them in a single layer on a parchment-lined roasting sheet.
- ❖ Roast the carrots in the preheated oven for about 20 minutes, until crisp-tender.
- ❖ Add the roasted carrots, ginger and milk to your food processor; puree the ingredients until everything is well blended.
- ❖ Enjoy

66) ONLY MEDITERRANEAN-STYLE ROASTED ARTICHOKES

Preparation Time: 50 minutes | | **Servings: 4**

Ingredients:

- ✓ 4 artichokes, trimmed, tough outer leaves and chokes removed, halved
- ✓ 2 lemons, freshly squeezed
- ✓ 4 tbsp extra-virgin olive oil
- ✓ 4 cloves garlic, chopped
- ✓ 1 tsp fresh rosemary
- ✓ 1 tsp fresh basil
- ✓ 1 tsp fresh parsley
- ✓ 1 tsp fresh oregano
- ✓ Flaky sea salt and ground black pepper, to taste
- ✓ 1 tsp red pepper flakes
- ✓ 1 tsp paprika

Directions:

- ❖ Start by preheating your oven to 395 degrees F. Rub the lemon juice all over the entire surface of your artichokes.
- ❖ In a small mixing bowl, thoroughly combine the garlic with herbs and spices
- ❖ Place the artichoke halves in a parchment-lined baking dish, cut-side-up. Brush the artichokes evenly with the olive oil. Fill the cavities with the garlic/herb mixture.
- ❖ Bake for about 20 minutes. Now, cover them with aluminum foil and bake for a further 30 minutes. Serve warm and enjoy

67) ASIAN THAI-STYLE BRAISED KALE

Preparation Time: 10 minutes | | **Servings: 4**

Ingredients:

- ✓ 1 cup water
- ✓ 1 ½ pounds kale, tough stems and ribs removed, torn into pieces
- ✓ 2 tbsp sesame oil
- ✓ 1 tsp fresh garlic, pressed
- ✓ 1 tsp ginger, peeled and minced
- ✓ 1 Thai chili, chopped
- ✓ 1/2 tsp turmeric powder
- ✓ 1/2 cup coconut milk
- ✓ Kosher salt and ground black pepper, to taste

Directions:

- ❖ In a large saucepan, bring the water to a rapid boil. Add in the kale and let it cook until bright, about 3 minutes. Drain, rinse and squeeze dry.
- ❖ Wipe the saucepan with paper towels and preheat the sesame oil over a moderate heat. Once hot, cook the garlic, ginger and chili for approximately 1 minute or so, until fragrant.
- ❖ Add in the kale and turmeric powder and continue to cook for a further 1 minute or until heated through.
- ❖ Gradually pour in the coconut milk, salt and black pepper; continue to simmer until the liquid has thickened. Taste, adjust the seasonings and serve hot. Enjoy

68) SPECIAL SILKY KOHLRABI PUREE

Preparation Time: 30 minutes		Servings: 4

Ingredients:

- ✓ 1 ½ pounds kohlrabi, peeled and cut into pieces
- ✓ 4 tbsp vegan butter
- ✓ Sea salt and freshly ground black pepper, to taste
- ✓ 1/2 tsp cumin seeds
- ✓ 1/2 tsp coriander seeds
- ✓ 1/2 cup soy milk
- ✓ 1 tsp fresh dill
- ✓ 1 tsp fresh parsley

Directions:

- ❖ Cook the kohlrabi in boiling salted water until soft, about 30 minutes; drain.
- ❖ Puree the kohlrabi with the vegan butter, salt, black pepper, cumin seeds and coriander seeds.
- ❖ Puree the ingredients with an immersion blender, gradually adding the milk. Top with fresh dill and parsley. Enjoy

69) TASTY CREAMY SAUTÉED SPINACH

Preparation Time: 15 minutes		Servings: 4

Ingredients:

- ✓ 2 tbsp vegan butter
- ✓ 1 onion, chopped
- ✓ 1 tsp garlic, minced
- ✓ 1 ½ cups vegetable broth
- ✓ 2 pounds spinach, torn into pieces
- ✓ Sea salt and ground black pepper, to taste
- ✓ 1/4 tsp dried dill
- ✓ 1/4 tsp mustard seeds
- ✓ 1/2 tsp celery seeds
- ✓ 1 tsp cayenne pepper
- ✓ 1/2 cup oat milk

Directions:

- ❖ In a saucepan, melt the vegan butter over medium-high heat.
- ❖ Then, sauté the onion for about 3 minutes or until tender and translucent. Then, sauté the garlic for about 1 minute until aromatic.
- ❖ Add in the broth and spinach and bring to a boil.
- ❖ Turn the heat to a simmer. Add in the spices and continue to cook for 5 minutes longer.
- ❖ Add in the milk and continue to cook for 5 minutes more. Enjoy

70) TORTILLA MEXICAN-STYLE SOUP

Preparation Time: 40 minutes		Servings: 4

Ingredients:

- ✓ 1 (14.5-oz) can diced tomatoes
- ✓ 1 (4-oz) can green chiles, chopped
- ✓ 2 tbsp olive oil
- ✓ 1 cup canned sweet corn
- ✓ 1 red onion, chopped
- ✓ 2 garlic cloves, minced
- ✓ 2 jalapeño peppers, sliced
- ✓ 4 cups vegetable broth
- ✓ 8 oz seitan, cut into ¼-inch strips
- ✓ Salt and black pepper to taste
- ✓ ¼ cup chopped fresh cilantro
- ✓ 3 tbsp fresh lime juice
- ✓ 4 corn tortillas, cut into strips
- ✓ 1 ripe avocado, chopped

Directions:

- ❖ Preheat oven to 350 F. Heat the oil in a pot over medium heat. Place sweet corn, garlic, jalapeño, and onion and cook for 5 minutes. Stir in broth, seitan, tomatoes, canned chiles, salt, and pepper. Bring to a boil, then lower the heat and simmer for 20 minutes. Put in the cilantro and lime juice, stir. Adjust the seasoning.
- ❖ Meanwhile, arrange the tortilla strips on a baking sheet and bake for 8 minutes until crisp. Serve the soup into bowls and top with tortilla strips and avocado

71) HOT BEAN SPICY SOUP

Preparation Time: 40 minutes		Servings: 4

Ingredients:

- ✓ 2 tbsp olive oil
- ✓ 1 medium onion, chopped
- ✓ 2 large garlic cloves, minced
- ✓ 1 carrot, chopped
- ✓ 1 (15.5-oz) can cannellini beans, drained
- ✓ 5 cups vegetable broth
- ✓ ¼ tsp crushed red pepper
- ✓ Salt and black pepper to taste
- ✓ 3 cups chopped baby spinach

Directions:

❖ Heat oil in a pot over medium heat. Place in carrot, onion, and garlic and cook for 3 minutes. Put in beans, broth, red pepper, salt, and black pepper and stir. Bring to a boil, then lower the heat and simmer for 25 minutes. Stir in baby spinach and cook for 5 minutes until the spinach wilts. Serve warm

72) SPECIAL MUSHROOM RICE WINE SOUP

Preparation Time: 25 minutes		Servings: 4

Ingredients:

- ✓ 2 tbsp olive oil
- ✓ 4 green onions, chopped
- ✓ 1 carrot, chopped
- ✓ 8 oz shiitake mushrooms, sliced
- ✓ 3 tbsp rice wine
- ✓ 2 tbsp soy sauce
- ✓ 4 cups vegetable broth
- ✓ Salt and black pepper to taste
- ✓ 2 tbsp parsley, chopped

Directions:

❖ Heat the oil in a pot over medium heat. Place the green onions and carrot and cook for 5 minutes.

❖ Stir in mushrooms, rice wine, soy sauce, broth, salt, and pepper. Bring to a boil, then lower the heat and simmer for 15 minutes. Top with parsley and serve warm

73) TASTY BEAN TANGY TOMATO SOUP

Preparation Time: 30 minutes		Servings: 5

Ingredients:

- ✓ 2 tsp olive oil
- ✓ 1 onion, chopped
- ✓ 2 garlic cloves, minced
- ✓ 1 cup mushrooms, chopped
- ✓ Sea salt to taste
- ✓ 1 tbsp dried basil
- ✓ ½ tbsp dried oregano
- ✓ 1 (19-oz) can diced tomatoes
- ✓ 1 (14-oz) can kidney beans, drained
- ✓ 5 cups water
- ✓ 2 cups chopped mustard greens

Directions:

❖ Heat the oil in a pot over medium heat. Place in the onion, garlic, mushrooms, and salt and cook for 5 minutes. Stir in basil and oregano, tomatoes, and beans. Pour in water and stir. Simmer for 20 minutes and add in mustard greens; cook for 5 minutes until greens soften. Serve immediately

74) Easy Spinach and Potato Soup

Preparation Time: 55 minutes		Servings: 4

Ingredients:

- ✓ 2 tbsp olive oil
- ✓ 1 onion, chopped
- ✓ 2 garlic cloves, minced
- ✓ 4 cups vegetable broth
- ✓ 2 russet potatoes, cubed
- ✓ ½ tsp dried oregano
- ✓ ¼ tsp crushed red pepper
- ✓ 1 bay leaf
- ✓ Salt to taste
- ✓ 4 cups chopped spinach
- ✓ 1 cup green lentils, rinsed

Directions:

- ❖ Warm the oil in a pot over medium heat. Place the onion and garlic and cook covered for 5 minutes. Stir in broth, potatoes, oregano, red pepper, bay leaf, lentils, and salt. Bring to a boil, then lower the heat and simmer uncovered for 30 minutes. Add in spinach and cook for another 5 minutes. Discard the bay leaf and serve immediately

75) MEXICAN BEAN TURMERIC SOUP

Preparation Time: 50 minutes		Servings: 6

Ingredients:

- ✓ 3 tbsp olive oil
- ✓ 1 onion, chopped
- ✓ 2 carrots, chopped
- ✓ 1 sweet potato, chopped
- ✓ 1 yellow bell pepper, chopped
- ✓ 2 garlic cloves, minced
- ✓ 4 tomatoes, chopped
- ✓ 6 cups vegetable broth
- ✓ 1 bay leaf
- ✓ Salt to taste
- ✓ 1 tsp ground cayenne pepper
- ✓ 1 (15.5-oz) can white beans, drained
- ✓ ⅓ cup whole-wheat pasta
- ✓ ¼ tsp turmeric

Directions:

- ❖ Heat the oil in a pot over medium heat. Place onion, carrots, sweet potato, bell pepper, and garlic. Cook for 5 minutes. Add in tomatoes, broth, bay leaf, salt, and cayenne pepper. Stir and bring to a boil. Lower the heat and simmer for 10 minutes. Put in white beans and simmer for 15 more minutes.
- ❖ Cook the pasta in a pot with boiling salted water and turmeric for 8-10 minutes, until pasta is al dente. Strain and transfer to the soup. Discard the bay leaf. Spoon into a bowl and serve

76) TROPICAL COCONUT ARUGULA SOUP

Preparation Time: 30 minutes		Servings: 4

Ingredients:

- ✓ 1 tsp coconut oil
- ✓ 1 onion, diced
- ✓ 2 cups green beans
- ✓ 4 cups water
- ✓ 1 cup arugula, chopped
- ✓ 1 tbsp fresh mint, chopped
- ✓ Sea salt and black pepper to taste
- ✓ ¾ cup coconut milk

Directions:

- ❖ Place a pot over medium heat and heat the coconut oil. Add in the onion and sauté for 5 minutes. Pour in green beans and water. Bring to a boil, lower the heat and stir in arugula, mint, salt, and pepper. Simmer for 10 minutes. Stir in coconut milk. Transfer to a food processor and blitz the soup until smooth. Serve

77) AUTHENTIC LENTIL SOUP WITH SWISS CHARD

Preparation Time: 25 minutes		Servings: 5

Ingredients:

- ✓ 2 tbsp olive oil
- ✓ 1 white onion, chopped
- ✓ 1 tsp garlic, minced
- ✓ 2 large carrots, chopped
- ✓ 1 parsnip, chopped
- ✓ 2 stalks celery, chopped
- ✓ 2 bay leaves

- ✓ 1/2 tsp dried thyme
- ✓ 1/4 tsp ground cumin
- ✓ 5 cups roasted vegetable broth
- ✓ 1 ¼ cups brown lentils, soaked overnight and rinsed
- ✓ 2 cups Swiss chard, torn into pieces

Directions:

- ❖ In a heavy-bottomed pot, heat the olive oil over a moderate heat. Now, sauté the vegetables along with the spices for about 3 minutes until they are just tender.
- ❖ Add in the vegetable broth and lentils, bringing it to a boil. Immediately turn the heat to a simmer and add in the bay leaves. Let it cook for about 15 minutes or until lentils are tender.
- ❖ Add in the Swiss chard, cover and let it simmer for 5 minutes more or until the chard wilts.
- ❖ Serve in individual bowls and enjoy

78) SPECIAL GREEN BEAN CREAM SALAD WITH PINE NUTS

Preparation Time: 10 minutes + chilling time		Servings: 5

Ingredients:

- ✓ 1 ½ pounds green beans, trimmed
- ✓ 2 medium tomatoes, diced
- ✓ 2 bell peppers, seeded and diced
- ✓ 4 tbsp shallots, chopped
- ✓ 1/2 cup pine nuts, roughly chopped

- ✓ 1/2 cup vegan mayonnaise
- ✓ 1 tbsp deli mustard
- ✓ 2 tbsp fresh basil, chopped
- ✓ 2 tbsp fresh parsley, chopped
- ✓ 1/2 tsp red pepper flakes, crushed
- ✓ Sea salt and freshly ground black pepper, to taste

Directions:

- ❖ Boil the green beans in a large saucepan of salted water until they are just tender or about 2 minutes.
- ❖ Drain and let the beans cool completely; then, transfer them to a salad bowl. Toss the beans with the remaining ingredients.
- ❖ Taste and adjust the seasonings. Enjoy

79) EASY KALE CANNELLINI BEAN SOUP

Preparation Time: 25 minutes		Servings: 5

Ingredients:

- ✓ 1 tbsp olive oil
- ✓ 1/2 tsp ginger, minced
- ✓ 1/2 tsp cumin seeds
- ✓ 1 red onion, chopped
- ✓ 1 carrot, trimmed and chopped
- ✓ 1 parsnip, trimmed and chopped

- ✓ 2 garlic cloves, minced
- ✓ 5 cups vegetable broth
- ✓ 12 ounces Cannellini beans, drained
- ✓ 2 cups kale, torn into pieces
- ✓ Sea salt and ground black pepper, to taste

Directions:

- ❖ In a heavy-bottomed pot, heat the olive over medium-high heat. Now, sauté the ginger and cumin for 1 minute or so.
- ❖ Now, add in the onion, carrot and parsnip; continue sautéing an additional 3 minutes or until the vegetables are just tender.
- ❖ Add in the garlic and continue to sauté for 1 minute or until aromatic.
- ❖ Then, pour in the vegetable broth and bring to a boil. Immediately reduce the heat to a simmer and let it cook for 10 minutes.
- ❖ Fold in the Cannellini beans and kale; continue to simmer until the kale wilts and everything is thoroughly heated. Season with salt and pepper to taste.
- ❖ Ladle into individual bowls and serve hot. Enjoy

80) DELICIOUS MUSHROOM SOUP WITH HEARTY CREAM

Preparation Time: 15 minutes		Servings: 5

Ingredients:

- ✓ 2 tbsp soy butter
- ✓ 1 large shallot, chopped
- ✓ 20 ounces Cremini mushrooms, sliced
- ✓ 2 cloves garlic, minced
- ✓ 4 tbsp flaxseed meal
- ✓ 5 cups vegetable broth
- ✓ 1 1/3 cups full-fat coconut milk
- ✓ 1 bay leaf
- ✓ Sea salt and ground black pepper, to taste

Directions:

- ❖ In a stockpot, melt the vegan butter over medium-high heat. Once hot, cook the shallot for about 3 minutes until tender and fragrant.
- ❖ Add in the mushrooms and garlic and continue cooking until the mushrooms have softened. Add in the flaxseed meal and continue to cook for 1 minute or so.
- ❖ Add in the remaining ingredients. Let it simmer, covered and continue to cook for 5 to 6 minutes more until your soup has thickened slightly.
- ❖ Enjoy

81) ITALIAN-STYLE AUTHENTIC PANZANELLA SALAD

Preparation Time: 35 minutes		Servings: 3

Ingredients:

- ✓ 3 cups artisan bread, broken into 1-inch cubes
- ✓ 3/4-pound asparagus, trimmed and cut into bite-sized pieces
- ✓ 4 tbsp extra-virgin olive oil
- ✓ 1 red onion, chopped
- ✓ 2 tbsp fresh lime juice
- ✓ 1 tsp deli mustard
- ✓ 2 medium heirloom tomatoes, diced
- ✓ 2 cups arugula
- ✓ 2 cups baby spinach
- ✓ 2 Italian peppers, seeded and sliced
- ✓ Sea salt and ground black pepper, to taste

Directions:

- ❖ Arrange the bread cubes on a parchment-lined baking sheet. Bake in the preheated oven at 310 degrees F for about 20 minutes, rotating the baking sheet twice during the baking time; reserve.
- ❖ Turn the oven to 420 degrees F and toss the asparagus with 1 tbsp of olive oil. Roast the asparagus for about 15 minutes or until crisp-tender.
- ❖ Toss the remaining ingredients in a salad bowl; top with the roasted asparagus and toasted bread.
- ❖ Enjoy

Chapter 4.   DESSERTS

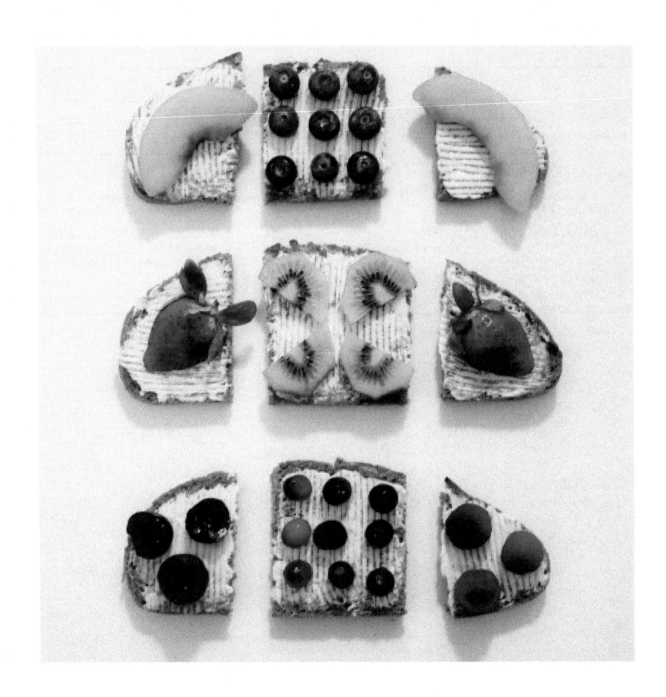

82) EVERYDAY BAKED APPLES FILLED WITH NUTS

Preparation Time: 35 minutes + cooling time		Servings: 4

Ingredients:

- ✓ 4 gala apples
- ✓ 3 tbsp pure maple syrup
- ✓ 4 tbsp almond flour
- ✓ 6 tbsp pure date sugar
- ✓ 6 tbsp plant butter, cold and cubed
- ✓ 1 cup chopped mixed nuts

Directions:

- ❖ Preheat the oven the 400 F.
- ❖ Slice off the top of the apples and use a melon baller or spoon to scoop out the cores of the apples. In a bowl, mix the maple syrup, almond flour, date sugar, butter, and nuts. Spoon the mixture into the apples and then bake in the oven for 25 minutes or until the nuts are golden brown on top and the apples soft. Remove the apples from the oven, allow cooling, and serve

83) SUMMER MINT ICE CREAM

Preparation Time: 10 minutes + chilling time		Servings: 4

Ingredients:

- ✓ 2 avocados, pitted
- ✓ 1 ¼ cups coconut cream
- ✓ ½ tsp vanilla extract
- ✓ 2 tbsp erythritol
- ✓ 2 tsp chopped mint leaves

Directions:

- ❖ Into a blender, spoon the avocado pulps, pour in the coconut cream, vanilla extract, erythritol, and mint leaves. Process until smooth. Pour the mixture into your ice cream maker and freeze according to the manufacturer's instructions. When ready, remove and scoop the ice cream into bowls. Serve

84) TASTY CARDAMOM COCONUT FAT BOMBS

Preparation Time: 10 minutes		Servings: 6

Ingredients:

- ✓ ½ cup grated coconut
- ✓ 3 oz plant butter, softened
- ✓ ¼ tsp green cardamom powder
- ✓ ½ tsp vanilla extract
- ✓ ¼ tsp cinnamon powder

Directions:

- ❖ Pour the grated coconut into a skillet and roast until lightly brown. Set aside to cool. In a bowl, combine butter, half of the coconut, cardamom, vanilla, and cinnamon. Form balls from the mixture and roll each one in the remaining coconut. Refrigerate until ready to serve

85) HUNGARIAN CINNAMON FAUX RICE PUDDING

Preparation Time: 25 minutes		Servings: 6

Ingredients:

- ✓ 1 ¼ cups coconut cream
- ✓ 1 tsp vanilla extract
- ✓ 1 tsp cinnamon powder
- ✓ 1 cup mashed tofu
- ✓ 2 oz fresh strawberries

Directions:

- ❖ Pour the coconut cream into a bowl and whisk until a soft peak forms. Mix in the vanilla and cinnamon. Lightly fold in the vegan cottage cheese and refrigerate for 10 to 15 minutes to set. Spoon into serving glasses, top with the strawberries and serve immediately

86) SWEET WHITE CHOCOLATE FUDGE

Preparation Time: 20 minutes + chilling time		**Servings: 6**

Ingredients:

- ✓ 2 cups coconut cream
- ✓ 1 tsp vanilla extract
- ✓ 3 oz plant butter
- ✓ 3 oz vegan white chocolate
- ✓ Swerve sugar for sprinkling

Directions:

❖ Pour coconut cream and vanilla into a saucepan and bring to a boil over medium heat, then simmer until reduced by half, 15 minutes. Stir in plant butter until the batter is smooth. Chop white chocolate into bits and stir in the cream until melted. Pour the mixture into a baking sheet; chill in the fridge for 3 hours. Cut into squares, sprinkle with swerve sugar, and serve

87) ITALIAN MACEDONIA SALAD WITH COCONUT AND PECANS

Preparation Time: 15 minutes + cooling time		**Servings: 4**

Ingredients:

- ✓ 1 cup pure coconut cream
- ✓ ½ tsp vanilla extract
- ✓ 2 bananas, cut into chunks
- ✓ 1 ½ cups coconut flakes
- ✓ 4 tbsp toasted pecans, chopped
- ✓ 1 cup pineapple tidbits, drained
- ✓ 1 (11-oz) can mandarin oranges
- ✓ ¾ cup maraschino cherries, stems removed

Directions:

❖ In a medium bowl, mix the coconut cream and vanilla extract until well combined.

❖ In a larger bowl, combine the bananas, coconut flakes, pecans, pineapple, oranges, and cherries until evenly distributed. Pour on the coconut cream mixture and fold well into the salad. Chill in the refrigerator for 1 hour and serve afterward

88) AUTHENTIC BERRY HAZELNUT TRIFLE

Preparation Time: 10 minutes		**Servings: 4**

Ingredients:

- ✓ 1 ½ ripe avocados
- ✓ ¾ cup coconut cream
- ✓ Zest and juice of ½ a lemon
- ✓ 1 tbsp vanilla extract
- ✓ 3 oz fresh strawberries
- ✓ 2 oz toasted hazelnuts

Directions:

❖ In a bowl, add avocado pulp, coconut cream, lemon zest and juice, and half of the vanilla extract. Mix with an immersion blender. Put the strawberries and remaining vanilla in another bowl and use a fork to mash the fruits. In a tall glass, alternate layering the cream and strawberry mixtures. Drop a few hazelnuts on each and serve the dessert immediately

89) VEGETARIAN AVOCADO TRUFFLES WITH CHOCOLATE COATING

Preparation Time: 5 minutes		**Servings: 6**

Ingredients:

- ✓ 1 ripe avocado, pitted
- ✓ ½ tsp vanilla extract
- ✓ ½ tsp lemon zest
- ✓ 5 oz dairy-free dark chocolate
- ✓ 1 tbsp coconut oil
- ✓ 1 tbsp unsweetened cocoa powder

Directions:

❖ Scoop the pulp of the avocado into a bowl and mix with the vanilla using an immersion blender. Stir in the lemon zest and a pinch of salt. Pour the chocolate and coconut oil into a safe microwave bowl and melt in the microwave for 1 minute. Add to the avocado mixture and stir. Allow cooling to firm up a bit. Form balls out of the mix. Roll each ball in the cocoa powder and serve immediately

90) DELICIOUS VANILLA BERRY TARTS

Preparation Time: 35 minutes + cooling time		Servings: 4

Ingredients:

- ✓ 4 tbsp flaxseed powder
- ✓ 1/3 cup whole-wheat flour
- ✓ ½ tsp salt
- ✓ ¼ cup plant butter, crumbled
- ✓ 3 tbsp pure malt syrup
- ✓ 6 oz cashew cream
- ✓ 6 tbsp pure date sugar
- ✓ ¾ tsp vanilla extract
- ✓ 1 cup mixed frozen berries

Directions:

- ❖ Preheat oven to 350 F and grease mini pie pans with cooking spray. In a bowl, mix flaxseed powder with 12 tbsp water and allow soaking for 5 minutes. In a large bowl, combine flour and salt. Add in butter and whisk until crumbly. Pour in the vegan "flax egg" and malt syrup and mix until smooth dough forms. Flatten the dough on a flat surface, cover with plastic wrap, and refrigerate for 1 hour.
- ❖ Dust a working surface with some flour, remove the dough onto the surface, and using a rolling pin, flatten the dough into a 1-inch diameter circle. Use a large cookie cutter, cut out rounds of the dough and fit into the pie pans. Use a knife to trim the edges of the pan. Lay a parchment paper on the dough cups, pour on some baking beans, and bake in the oven until golden brown, 15-20 minutes. Remove the pans from the oven, pour out the baking beans, and allow cooling. In a bowl, mix cashew cream, date sugar, and vanilla extract. Divide the mixture into the tart cups and top with berries. Serve

91) BEST HOMEMADE CHOCOLATES WITH COCONUT AND RAISINS

Preparation Time: 10 minutes + chilling time		Servings: 20

Ingredients:

- ✓ 1/2 cup cacao butter, melted
- ✓ 1/3 cup peanut butter
- ✓ 1/4 cup agave syrup
- ✓ A pinch of grated nutmeg
- ✓ A pinch of coarse salt
- ✓ 1/2 tsp vanilla extract
- ✓ 1 cup dried coconut, shredded
- ✓ 6 ounces dark chocolate, chopped
- ✓ 3 ounces raisins

Directions:

- ❖ Thoroughly combine all the ingredients, except for the chocolate, in a mixing bowl.
- ❖ Spoon the mixture into molds. Leave to set hard in a cool place.
- ❖ Melt the dark chocolate in your microwave. Pour in the melted chocolate until the fillings are covered. Leave to set hard in a cool place.
- ❖ Enjoy

92) SIMPLE MOCHA FUDGE

Preparation Time: 1 hour 10 minutes		Servings: 20

Ingredients:

- ✓ 1 cup cookies, crushed
- ✓ 1/2 cup almond butter
- ✓ 1/4 cup agave nectar
- ✓ 6 ounces dark chocolate, broken into chunks
- ✓ 1 tsp instant coffee
- ✓ A pinch of grated nutmeg
- ✓ A pinch of salt

Directions:

- ❖ Line a large baking sheet with parchment paper.
- ❖ Melt the chocolate in your microwave and add in the remaining ingredients; stir to combine well.
- ❖ Scrape the batter into a parchment-lined baking sheet. Place it in your freezer for at least 1 hour to set.
- ❖ Cut into squares and serve. Enjoy

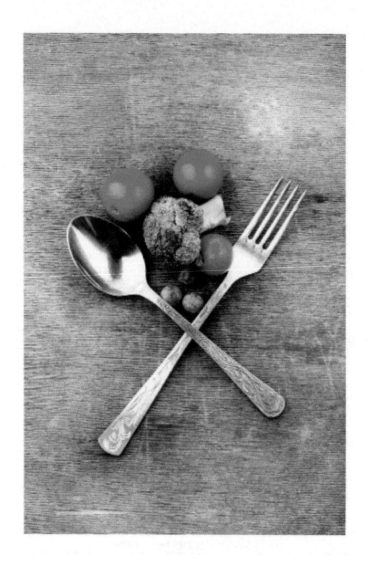

immagine

93) EAST ALMOND AND CHOCOLATE CHIP BARS

Preparation Time: 40 minutes		Servings: 10

Ingredients:

- ✓ 1/2 cup almond butter
- ✓ 1/4 cup coconut oil, melted
- ✓ 1/4 cup agave syrup
- ✓ 1 tsp vanilla extract
- ✓ 1/4 tsp sea salt
- ✓ 1/4 tsp grated nutmeg
- ✓ 1/2 tsp ground cinnamon
- ✓ 2 cups almond flour
- ✓ 1/4 cup flaxseed meal
- ✓ 1 cup vegan chocolate, cut into chunks
- ✓ 1 1/3 cups almonds, ground
- ✓ 2 tbsp cacao powder
- ✓ 1/4 cup agave syrup

Directions:

- ❖ In a mixing bowl, thoroughly combine the almond butter, coconut oil, 1/4 cup of agave syrup, vanilla, salt, nutmeg and cinnamon.
- ❖ Gradually stir in the almond flour and flaxseed meal and stir to combine. Add in the chocolate chunks and stir again.
- ❖ In a small mixing bowl, combine the almonds, cacao powder and agave syrup. Now, spread the ganache onto the cake. Freeze for about 30 minutes, cut into bars and serve well chilled. Enjoy

94) ALMOND BUTTER COOKIES

Preparation Time: 45 minutes		Servings: 10

Ingredients:

- ✓ 3/4 cup all-purpose flour
- ✓ 1/2 tsp baking soda
- ✓ 1/4 tsp kosher salt
- ✓ 1 flax egg
- ✓ 1/4 cup coconut oil, at room temperature
- ✓ 2 tbsp almond milk
- ✓ 1/2 cup brown sugar
- ✓ 1/2 cup almond butter
- ✓ 1/2 tsp ground cinnamon
- ✓ 1/2 tsp vanilla

Directions:

- ❖ In a mixing bowl, combine the flour, baking soda and salt.
- ❖ In another bowl, combine the flax egg, coconut oil, almond milk, sugar, almond butter, cinnamon and vanilla. Stir the wet mixture into the dry ingredients and stir until well combined.
- ❖ Place the batter in your refrigerator for about 30 minutes. Shape the batter into small cookies and arrange them on a parchment-lined cookie pan.
- ❖ Bake in the preheated oven at 350 degrees F for approximately 12 minutes. Transfer the pan to a wire rack to cool at room temperature. Enjoy

95) SUMMER RAW RASPBERRY CHEESECAKE

Preparation Time: 15 minutes + chilling time		Servings: 9

Ingredients:

- ✓ Crust:
- ✓ 2 cups almonds
- ✓ 1 cup fresh dates, pitted
- ✓ 1/4 tsp ground cinnamon
- ✓ Filling:
- ✓ 2 cups raw cashews, soaked overnight and drained
- ✓ 14 ounces blackberries, frozen
- ✓ 1 tbsp fresh lime juice
- ✓ 1/4 tsp crystallized ginger
- ✓ 1 can coconut cream
- ✓ 8 fresh dates, pitted

Directions:

- ❖ In your food processor, blend the crust ingredients until the mixture comes together; press the crust into a lightly oiled springform pan.
- ❖ Then, blend the filling layer until completely smooth. Spoon the filling onto the crust, creating a flat surface with a spatula.
- ❖ Transfer the cake to your freezer for about 3 hours. Store in your freezer.
- ❖ Garnish with organic citrus peel. Enjoy

96) EASY MINI LEMON TARTS

Preparation Time: 15 minutes + chilling time		Servings: 9

Ingredients:

- ✓ 1 cup cashews
- ✓ 1 cup dates, pitted
- ✓ 1/2 cup coconut flakes
- ✓ 1/2 tsp anise, ground
- ✓ 3 lemons, freshly squeezed
- ✓ 1 cup coconut cream
- ✓ 2 tbsp agave syrup

Directions:

- ❖ Brush a muffin tin with a nonstick cooking oil.
- ❖ Blend the cashews, dates, coconut and anise in your food processor or a high-speed blender. Press the crust into the peppered muffin tin.
- ❖ Then, blend the lemon, coconut cream and agave syrup. Spoon the cream into the muffin tin.
- ❖ Store in your freezer. Enjoy

97) EXOTIC COCONUT BLONDIES WITH RAISINS

Preparation Time: 30 minutes		Servings: 9

Ingredients:

- ✓ 1 cup coconut flour
- ✓ 1 cup all-purpose flour
- ✓ 1/2 tsp baking powder
- ✓ 1/4 tsp salt
- ✓ 1 cup desiccated coconut, unsweetened
- ✓ 3/4 cup vegan butter, softened
- ✓ 1 ½ cups brown sugar
- ✓ 3 tbsp applesauce
- ✓ 1/2 tsp vanilla extract
- ✓ 1/2 tsp ground anise
- ✓ 1 cup raisins, soaked for 15 minutes

Directions:

- ❖ Start by preheating your oven to 350 degrees F. Brush a baking pan with a nonstick cooking oil.
- ❖ Thoroughly combine the flour, baking powder, salt and coconut. In another bowl, mix the butter, sugar, applesauce, vanilla and anise. Stir the butter mixture into the dry ingredients; stir to combine well.
- ❖ Fold in the raisins. Press the batter into the prepared baking pan.
- ❖ Bake for approximately 25 minutes or until it is set in the middle. Place the cake on a wire rack to cool slightly.
- ❖ Enjoy

98) SIMPLE CHOCOLATE SQUARES

Preparation Time: 1 hour 10 minutes		Servings: 20

Ingredients:

- ✓ 1 cup cashew butter
- ✓ 1 cup almond butter
- ✓ 1/4 cup coconut oil, melted
- ✓ 1/4 cup raw cacao powder
- ✓ 2 ounces dark chocolate
- ✓ 4 tbsp agave syrup
- ✓ 1 tsp vanilla paste
- ✓ 1/4 tsp ground cinnamon
- ✓ 1/4 tsp ground cloves

Directions:

- ❖ Process all the ingredients in your blender until uniform and smooth.
- ❖ Scrape the batter into a parchment-lined baking sheet. Place it in your freezer for at least 1 hour to set.
- ❖ Cut into squares and serve. Enjoy

99) DELICIOUS CHOCOLATE AND RAISIN COOKIE BARS

Preparation Time: 40 minutes		Servings: 10

Ingredients:

- ✓ 1/2 cup peanut butter, at room temperature
- ✓ 1 cup agave syrup
- ✓ 1 tsp pure vanilla extract
- ✓ 1/4 tsp kosher salt
- ✓ 2 cups almond flour
- ✓ 1 tsp baking soda
- ✓ 1 cup raisins
- ✓ 1 cup vegan chocolate, broken into chunks

Directions:

- ❖ In a mixing bowl, thoroughly combine the peanut butter, agave syrup, vanilla and salt.
- ❖ Gradually stir in the almond flour and baking soda and stir to combine. Add in the raisins and chocolate chunks and stir again.
- ❖ Freeze for about 30 minutes and serve well chilled. Enjoy

100) TASTY ALMOND GRANOLA BARS

Preparation Time: 25 minutes | | **Servings: 12**

Ingredients:

- ✓ 1/2 cup spelt flour
- ✓ 1/2 cup oat flour
- ✓ 1 cup rolled oats
- ✓ 1 tsp baking powder
- ✓ 1/2 tsp cinnamon
- ✓ 1/2 tsp ground cardamom
- ✓ 1/4 tsp freshly grated nutmeg
- ✓ 1/8 tsp kosher salt
- ✓ 1 cup almond milk
- ✓ 3 tbsp agave syrup
- ✓ 1/2 cup peanut butter
- ✓ 1/2 cup applesauce
- ✓ 1/2 tsp pure almond extract
- ✓ 1/2 tsp pure vanilla extract
- ✓ 1/2 cup almonds, slivered

Directions:

- ❖ Begin by preheating your oven to 350 degrees F.
- ❖ In a mixing bowl, thoroughly combine the flour, oats, baking powder and spices. In another bowl, combine the wet ingredients.
- ❖ Then, stir the wet mixture into the dry ingredients; mix to combine well. Fold in the slivered almonds.
- ❖ Scrape the batter mixture into a parchment-lined baking pan. Bake in the preheated oven for about 20 minutes. Let it cool on a wire rack. Cut into bars and enjoy

101) TROPICAL COCONUT COOKIES

Preparation Time: 40 minutes | | **Servings: 10**

Ingredients:

- ✓ 1/2 cup oat flour
- ✓ 1/2 cup all-purpose flour
- ✓ 1/2 tsp baking soda
- ✓ A pinch of salt
- ✓ 1/4 tsp grated nutmeg
- ✓ 1/2 tsp ground cloves
- ✓ 1/2 tsp ground cinnamon
- ✓ 4 tbsp coconut oil
- ✓ 2 tbsp oat milk
- ✓ 1/2 cup coconut sugar
- ✓ 1/2 cup coconut flakes, unsweetened

Directions:

- ❖ In a mixing bowl, combine the flour, baking soda and spices.
- ❖ In another bowl, combine the coconut oil, oat milk, sugar and coconut. Stir the wet mixture into the dry ingredients and stir until well combined.
- ❖ Place the batter in your refrigerator for about 30 minutes. Shape the batter into small cookies and arrange them on a parchment-lined cookie pan.
- ❖ Bake in the preheated oven at 330 degrees F for approximately 10 minutes. Transfer the pan to a wire rack to cool at room temperature. Enjoy

102) HEALTHY RAW WALNUT AND BERRY CAKE

Preparation Time: 10 minutes + chilling time | | **Servings: 8**

Ingredients:

- ✓ Crust:
- ✓ 1 ½ cups walnuts, ground
- ✓ 2 tbsp maple syrup
- ✓ 1/4 cup raw cacao powder
- ✓ 1/4 tsp ground cinnamon
- ✓ A pinch of coarse salt
- ✓ A pinch of freshly grated nutmeg
- ✓ Berry layer:
- ✓ 6 cups mixed berries
- ✓ 2 frozen bananas
- ✓ 1/2 cup agave syrup

Directions:

- ❖ In your food processor, blend the crust ingredients until the mixture comes together; press the crust into a lightly oiled baking pan.
- ❖ Then, blend the berry layer. Spoon the berry layer onto the crust, creating a flat surface with a spatula.
- ❖ Transfer the cake to your freezer for about 3 hours. Store in your freezer. Enjoy

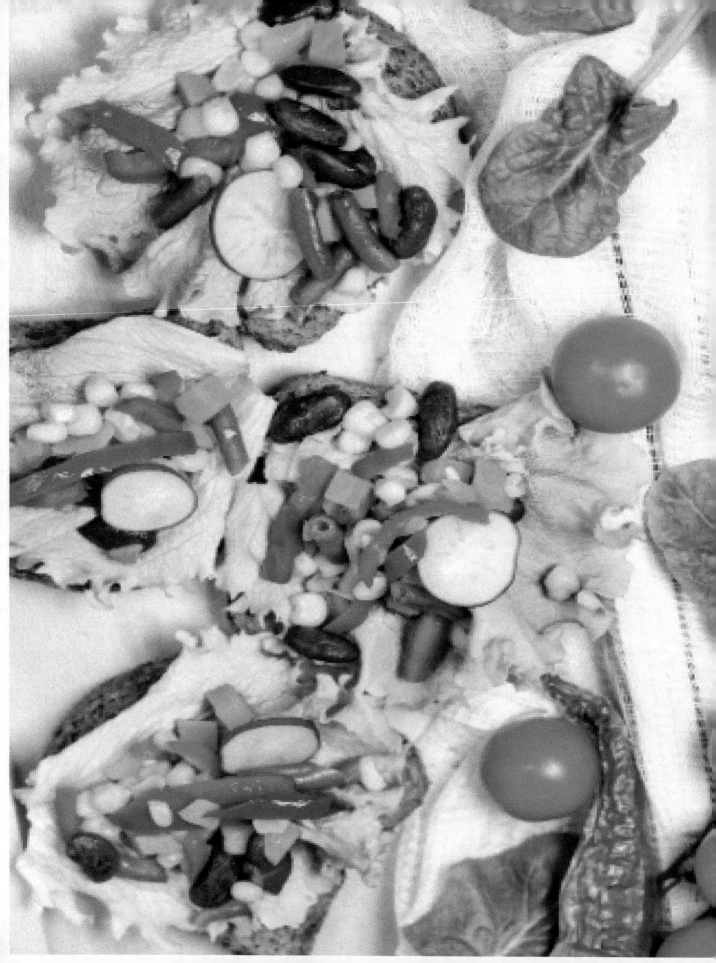

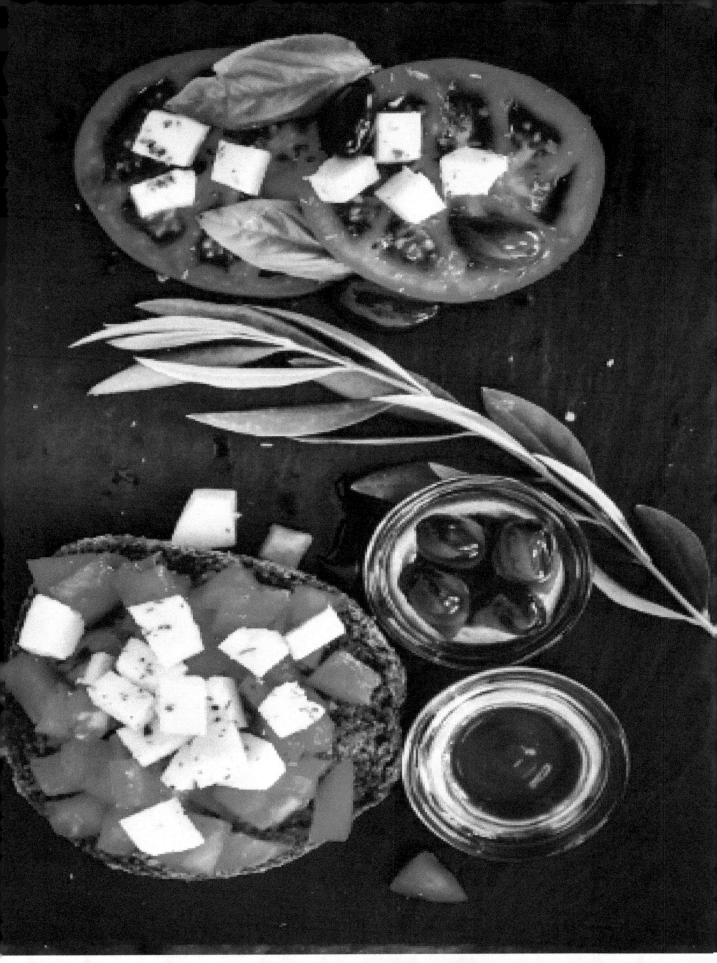

Bibliography

FROM THE SAME AUTHOR

THE VEGETARIAN DIET *Cookbook* - 100+ Easy-to-Follow Recipes for Beginners! TASTE Yourself with the Most Vibrant Plant-Based Cuisine Meals!

THE VEGETARIAN DIET FOR ATHLETES *Cookbook* - The Best Recipes for Athletic Performance and Muscle Growth! More Than 100 High-Protein Plant-Based Meals to Maintain a Perfect Body!

THE VEGETARIAN DIET FOR BEGINNERS *Cookbook* - 100+ Super Easy Recipes to Start a Healthier Lifestyle! The Best Recipes You Need to Jump into the Tastiest Plant-Based World!

THE VEGETARIAN DIET FOR MEN *Cookbook* - The Best 100 Recipes to Stay FIT! Sculpt Your Abs Before Summer with the Healthiest Plant-Based Meals!

THE VEGETARIAN DIET FOR WOMEN *Cookbook* - The Best 100 recipes to stay TONE and HEALTHY! Reboot your Metabolism before Summer with the Tastiest and Lightest Plant-Based Meals!

THE VEGETARIAN DIET FOR KIDS *Cookbook* - The Best 100 recipes for children, tested BY Kids FOR Kids! Jump into the Plant-Based World to Stay Healthy HAVING FUN!

THE VEGETARIAN DIET FOR WOMEN OVER 50 *Cookbook* - The Best Plant-Based Recipes to Restart Your Metabolism! Maintain the Right Hormonal Balance and Lose Weight with More Than 100 Light and Healthy Recipes!

THE VEGETARIAN DIET FOT MEN OVER 50 *Cookbook* - The Best Recipes to Restart Your Metabolism! Stay Healthy with More than 100 Easy and Mouthwatering Recipes!

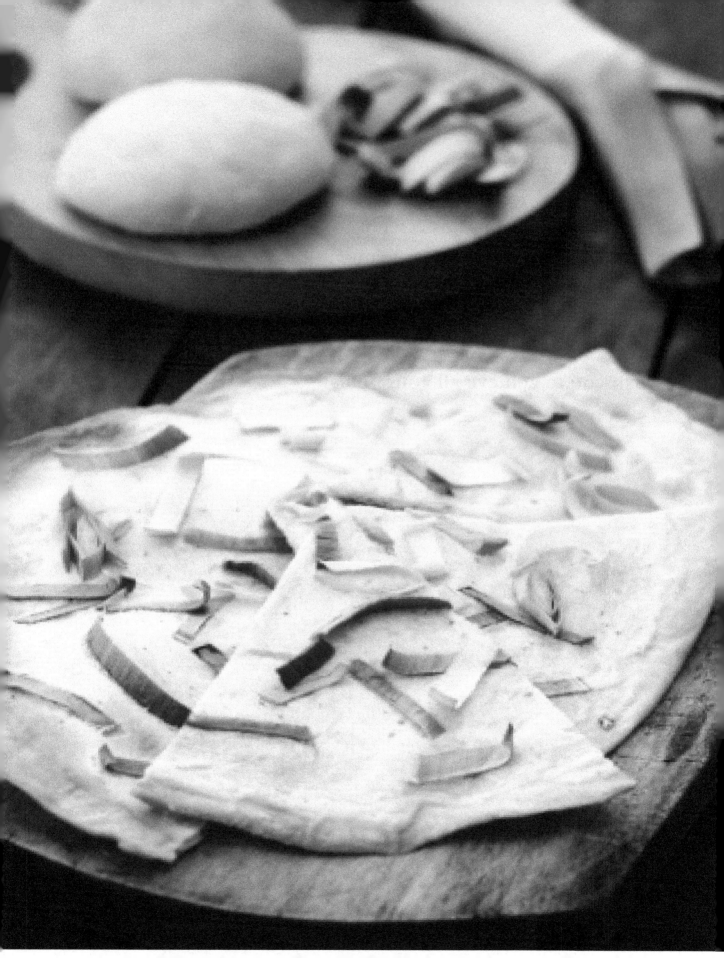

Conclusion

Thanks for reading "Vegetarian Diet for Beginners *Cookbook*"

Follow the right habits it is essential to have a healthy Lifestyle, and the Vegetarian diet is the best solution!

I hope you liked these Recipes!

I wish you to achieve all your goals!

Jocelyn Grant

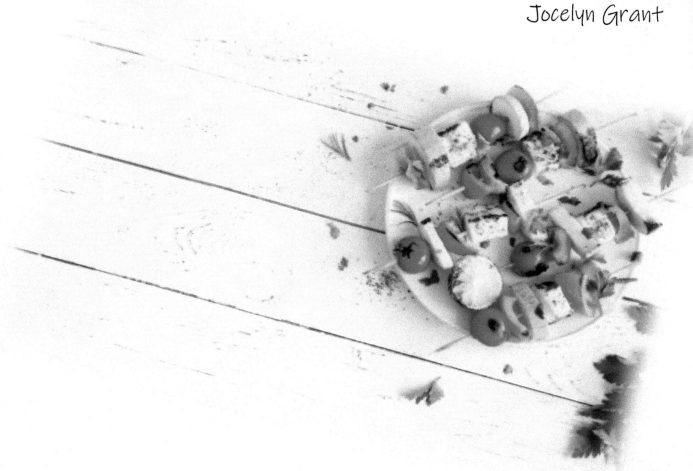

Lightning Source UK Ltd.
Milton Keynes UK
UKHW051438230421
382488UK00002B/131